GREED: SEX, MONEY, POWER, AND POLITICS

Edited by
Elizabeth Ronis, MSW, LCSW, BCD
and
Leslie Shaw, MBA, PhD,

IPBOOKS.net
International Psychoanalytic Books

A Division of International Psychoanalytic Media Group

Library of Congress Control number 2011934298

ISBN: 978-0-615-30910-1

GREED: SEX, MONEY, POWER, AND POLITICS

Contents

Contributors

Christopher Cutler, CFA, President of Manager Analysis Services, LLC [MAS], which advises investors in managing their portfolio of hedge fund investments. He founded MAS in 2003. From 1994 to 2003, Cutler worked at Deutsche Bank in New York in many capacities in its fixed income trading division. From 1988 to 1994, Cutler worked at the Federal Reserve Bank of New York as an emerging markets economist and a bank analyst. He graduated from The Uni-versity of Chicago in 1987 with a B.A. in Economics and from the NYU Stern School of Business in 1993 with an MBA in Finance. He is an active member of the New York Society of Securities Analysts, and had also chaired this Society's Alternative Investment Committee from 2005 to 2007.

Robert M. Galatzer-Levy, MD, Chicago child, adolescent, and adult analyst. A principal of Analytic Consultants, a firm that addresses business problems from a psychoanalytic viewpoint. Author of four books and over 100 papers and chapters; Faculty, University of Chicago and the Chicago Institute for Psychoanalysis. Current interests include nonlinear dynamics, clinical issues in psychoanalysis, psychology of law, and the application of psychoanalysis in the larger community.

Stephen Greenspan, PhD, Emeritus Professor of Educational Psychology at the University of Connecticut and Clinical Professor of Psychiatry at the University of Colorado. His scholarly focus is on social incompetence, and his forthcoming book is entitled *Anatomy of Foolishness*. In 2011, he received the John Jacobson Award for Critical Thinking from the American Psychological Association.

Lawrence Josephs, PhD, Professor, Derner Institute of Advanced Psychological Studies, Adelphi University; Editorial Boards, *International Journal of Psychoanalysis* and *Psychoanalysis and Psychotherapy.* Areas of interest: Superego functioning, infidelity and betrayal trauma, process and outcome research in psychoanalysis and psychotherapy, priming unconscious conflicts. Author, *Balancing Empathy and Interpretation.* (1995) and *Character Structure and the Organization of the Self* (1992).

Janice S. Lieberman, PhD, Training and Supervising Analyst, Faculty and Fellowship Chair, IPTAR; Editorial Board *JAPA*; Book Review Editor, *PANY Bulletin.* Author of *Body Talk: Looking and Being Looked at in Psychotherapy* (Jason Aronson 2000), and coauthor of *The Many Faces of Deceit: Omissions, Lies and Disguise in Psychotherapy* (Jason Aronson 1996). She has written on gender, body image,shame,greed and contemporary art from a psychoanalytic perspective.

Elliot Noma, PhD, Managing Director, Garrett Asset Management; founder of Garrett Asset Management, a systematic trading firm that uses technical systems to invest in futures, ETFs, and currencies. Consultant on a variety of financial issues involving portfolio management, hedge fund due diligence, trading systems, risk management, and operational due diligence. Former portfolio manager for the BTOP50 fund, a diversified portfolio of global macro, commodity, and managed futures programs. Ph.D in Mathematical Psychology in 1982 from The University of Michigan. Dr. Noma's research has been published in numerous industry journals and scholarly periodicals.

Arlene Kramer Richards, EdD, Training and Supervising Analyst, New York Freudian Society; member, APsaA and IPA, Author, *How to Get it Together When Your Parents are Coming Apart* (Random House Children's Books, 1976), and coeditor, *Fantasy Myth and Reality: Essays in Honor of Jacob Arlow* (IUP, 1988) and papers on female sexuality, perversion, and gambling.

Arnold D. Richards, MD, Training and Supervising Analyst, New York Psychoanalytic Institute, former Editor of *JAPA* (1994–2003), and *The American Psychoanalyst* (1989–1994); Faculty, Department of Psychiatry, NYU. Member, APA Division 39, Section I, New York Freudian Society, honorary member, Karen Horney Clinic and the New Jersey Psychoanalytic Society.

Elizabeth Ronis, LCSW, BCD. NPAP, Certified in Psychoanalysis, 1982; Member, Training Analyst, Supervisor, Former Treasurer, member of Training and Program Committees, Deptartment. of Psychiatry Adjunct Teaching Assistant, Mount Sinai School of Medicine; Symposium Co-Chair (2009–2011); Former Coordinator, Chinese-American Psychoanalytic Association (CAPA, 1996–2011); Training Analyst,

Supervisor Faculty, President, Vice President and Treasurer, Council of Psychoanalytic Therapists, Woodrow Wilson Teaching Fellowship; Member APA, Division 39; Former member NY Society of Security Analysts; Life member Art Students league; In private practice in NYC.

Jeffrey Stern, PhD, Faculty, Institute for Psychoanalysis, and University of Chicago. Lecturer on psychiatry, Shakespeare, and film. Published chapters in *Errant Selves: A Casebook of Misbehavior,* ed. by A. Goldberg, and *Transforming Lives: Analysts and Patients View the Power of Psychoanalytic Treatment,* ed. by J. Schachter; articles in *Shakespeare Quarterly, JAPA, Psychoanalytic Review, Psychoanalytic Psychology, Progress in Self Psychology, The International Journal of Psychoanalytic Self Psychology,* and *The Annual of Psychoanalysis,* of which he is Associate Editor.

Leslie Shaw, MBA, PhD, CORST graduate of core-training program, Chicago Psychoanalytic Institute. Experienced as organizational management consultant and project manager involving acquisitions, mergers, and management of staff transitions. Continues consulting, applied research in financial decision making, and teaching. Published "Long Term Capital Management and the Uncanny" in the *International Journal of Applied Psychoanalytic Studies* (2005), and " The Principal-Agent Relationship and Investment Decision-Making" in Behavioral Finance (1995), a CFA Institute Book in Continuing Education.

Christopher J. Topolewski, Esq., Principal and shareholder with West Capital Management, a registered investment advisory firm located in Philadelphia, PA. West Capital Management works with families and business owners to provide family office services to help accomplish their personal and financial goals. Chris received his Juris Doctorate from Villanova School of Law and graduated from Boston University School of Management with a BSBA in Finance.

Richard Tuch, MD, Training/Supervising Analyst, the New Center for Psychoanalysis in Los Angeles, and the Psychoanalytic Center of Califonia. Assistant Clinical Professor of Psychiatry, Geffen School of Medicine, UCLA. Recipient, Karl Menninger Memorial Award for Psychoanalytic Writing (1995) and the Edith Sabshin Teaching Award (2008). Frequent APsaA presenter, published in *IJP, JAPA,* and *Psychoanalytic Quarterly.* Author, *The Single*

Woman-Married Man Syndrome; Executive Editor, *Edinburgh International Encyclopedia of Psychoanalysis* (2006).

Bryant L. Welch, JD, PhD, Author of *State of Confusion: Political Manipulation and the Assault on the American Mind* (Thomas Dunne Books, St. Martin's Press, 2008). He organized the class action lawsuit Welch v. American Psychoanalytic Association that opened training in psychoanalysis around the country and also established the American Psychological Association Practice Directorate serving as its first executive director. He is a research associate graduate of the Washington Psychoanalytic Association and currently lives and practices psychology in San Francisco where he serves as Program Director for Clinical Psychology at the California Institute of Integral Studies (CIIS).

Mitchell Wilson, MD, Training and Supervising Analyst, San Francisco Center for Psychoanalysis and Psychotherapy. Awarded the Heinz Hartmann Memorial Lectureship at the New York Psychoanalytic Institute in 2002, the *JAPA* Journal Prize in 2003, and the Karl A. Menninger Memorial Award in 2005. He was formerly on the Editorial Board of *JAPA.* He has a psychoanalytic and supervisory practice in Berkeley, CA.

Kenneth Winarick, PhD, Past President, Director of Training, Training and Supervising Analyst, The American Institute for Psychoanalysis, Karen Horney Psychoanalytic Center. Past Director, Faculty, and Supervisor, The Psychological Internship Training Program of the Karen Horney Clinic. Graduate, Child and Adolescent Psychoanalytic Program of the New York Freudian Society

Peter Wolson, PhD, Training/Supervising Analyst and faculty, L.A. Institute and Society for Psychoanalytic Studies (LAISPS). Chair, Committee of Training Analysts; Founder of Confederation of Independent Psa. Societies; Past President & Director of Training, LAISPS; Resident Faculty, Wright Institute of L.A. Articles on adaptive grandiosity in artistic creativity & fatherhood, the existential dimension of psychoanalysis, analytic love, and op-ed pieces for the *Los Angeles Times, The Huffington Post,* and *Counterpunch.* In private practice, Beverly Hills, CA.

Symposium 2009 and Psychoanalytic Irony[1]

At the time of this writing it has been more than one year since *Symposium 2009: Money, Greed, Sex, Power and Politics* was held in New York City at Mount Sinai Medical Center. The impetus for the conference was the financial crisis, of course. The sheer number of psychoanalytic and psychiatric sponsoring organizations was remarkable. The entire professional field in New York seemed to be involved and there was even a sponsor from London. With limited exception, all of the speakers were psychoanalytic clinicians from different cities in the United States. The papers were superbly written and presented. Audience discussion was energized. The underlying emotional sense that Psychoanalysis was *The* Forum in which to understand such human crises was palpable. For Psychoanalysis, our day had come, so to speak. We could have predicted that a seething mass of desires would inevitably bring us to the brink. As you will see the clinical perspectives that are presented in this volume are near perfection. We have proven that Psychoanalysis is not dead because the world so obviously needs us. Unfortunately and with regret this brilliant Symposium came to a close before we were able to determine any therapeutic action for the future of the world or, even more realistically, for the place of Psychoanalysis within the future.

And so it is the purpose of this Foreword to set the stage for the presentation of the particular topics that were chosen for Symposium, 2009. Why do recent events, especially, convince Psychoanalysis ever more that its time is now? Psychoanalysis seems to have an uncanny sense about its capacity for insight regarding the topics of the Symposium. Yet the profession itself has been described as being in decline for at least three or four decades. The primary criticism is that we have not generated any new ideas during that long a period of time.[2] The Symposium 2009 was largely a discussion among psychoanalytic clinicians and for a psychoanalytically informed audience. Thus the clinical perspective in the majority of papers was of inherent interest. Nevertheless, it has been nearly two decades since Arnold Goldberg suggested that the clinical case might also be evocative of the problem of a developmental impasse within Psychoanalysis. "We need to ask where our field is in terms of having and pursuing a life of its own as well as experiencing developmental problems of its own". Goldberg wrote that the psychoanalytic enterprise is a closed system. One that is bounded by rules of behavior, its allegiance to its heroes, and its reliance on a theory that, in turn, derives from and insists upon a set of absolutes or fundamental assumptions. He called for an opening of the closed system that keeps psychoanalysis within its own prison. And he hoped for radical changes that would allow psychoanalysis to evolve over time and in an unpredictable manner.[3] Goldberg's view has been supported by philosophical trends[4] and also by the newer ideas in neuroscience.

So how might this particular Symposium 2009 become remembered and cited as an occasion on which the papers and discussion of the event provided a portal into the structure of psychoanalysis that has sustained its own hermetic seal for so many decades?

My suggestion is that this Foreword becomes an entry into the psychoanalytic discussion that was the Symposium, 2009. So that at the end of this Foreword you, the reader, will be joining us as we were, in a written replay of the presentation of Symposium 2009 as it occurred. But as your unique prelude to that event there is some history that is not "of psychoanalysis" so much as it is "of the world", albeit very much around the history of psychoanalysis, almost since its inception. A description of the particular history that has been "around psychoanalysis" will next be presented. And then you are invited to join in an ongoing conversation that we will be able to say began on the occasion of New York Symposium 2009. How the conversation will evolve or where it will take us in the future is unpredictable. Therefore, "welcome" to Symposium 2009 on Greed, Sex, Money, Power and Politics. Before we hear from our speakers and their formal papers there is some history that has been around psychoanalysis for decades. It is inevitably and directly linked to the topics of interest for this Symposium; i.e., "Greed, Sex, Money, Power and Politics."

A Historic Irony

In 2002 an award winning television producer for the BBC, Adam Curtis, produced a four part documentary series that was titled "Century of the Self."[5] It received rave critical reviews and, for a time in 2005, the complete four-part film was played at a Greenwich Village movie theater in New York. The film came to be because the journalist producer Curtis found what he believed to be intriguing information that Sigmund Freud's nephew, Edward Bernays (1891–1995) had invented the field of public relations, specifically using his uncle's ideas about human beings and human nature. Curtis became intrigued enough to begin researching how Freud's ideas became used generally in social and political ways, not in any way telling the history of psychoanalysis but the history of how psychoanalytic ideas, at least via Freud's nephew Bernays, became applied and, according to the film, continue to be applied today. Part I of the documentary chronicles Edward Bernays's beginning career and his extraordinary link to his uncle Sigmund.

Bernays's father, Ely, was the brother of Freud's wife and Edward's mother was Sigmund Freud's sister, Anna. Ely and Anna Bernays came to America at the turn of the century. They left a couple of young daughters in Austria with Freud and Freud's parents until Ely became established in the new country and could afford to bring them. But the Bernayses brought their only son Edward along with them when they came to America. Edward (Eddie) grew up in New York. Nevertheless Eddie had ample opportunity to remain in touch with the family and his uncle, over the years. They often visited on holidays in Europe. Then in 1913 when Eddie was twenty-two he arranged to deliver a young boy to his mother, in Paris, in exchange for ship's fare. After delivering the boy Eddie immediately went to Carlsbad, in (what is now) the Czech Republic, where the Freud family was vacationing. On this trip Eddie and his uncle Sigmund took long walks in the woods. Years later Eddie recalled Freud's "pleasant and easy attitude, his understanding sympathy, more candid and relaxed in his attitude to me than any other older man I had ever known". "It was as if two close friends were exchanging confidences instead of a famous uncle of fifty-seven and an unknown nephew of twenty-two".

Whatever the specifics of their conversation it was clear that when Eddie returned to New York in the fall of 1913 he was more taken than ever with the Viennese doctor's novel theories on how unconscious drives, dating to childhood, make people act the way they do. And Eddie was convinced that understanding the instincts and symbols that motivate an individual could help him shape the behavior of the masses.

Back in New York Eddie Bernays began his career as a press agent and promoter for visiting show business personalities on Broadway. He had famous clients including Caruso and Ziegfeld. Eddie was so good at his job that he was asked to join the War Department's Committee on Public Information, the propaganda arm of the US war effort. Following the armistice, Eddie was still a very young man, but so regarded that he accompanied Woodrow Wilson to Paris and the Peace Conference in Europe. Wilson's campaign at the Peace Conference was essentially that America had fought to help bring democracy to all of Europe. Wilson said that he would continue to work to make the world safe for democracy. Wilson and America were seen as an economic liberator of people.

Bernays was only in his twenties and he was stunned by the way the crowds in Paris heralded President Wilson. Eddie found himself thinking about the way that propaganda had been used to fight the war. He wondered if there might be a way to manage and alter the way that people made decisions. Could they be manipulated in peace time as well? While Bernays was on this trip to Paris he sent his Uncle Sigmund a gift box of Havana Cigars, which at the time were hard to get in Vienna. Upon return from Paris Bernays conducted a very successful campaign to promote re-employment of returning veterans. His effective use of publicity and the enlistment of civic groups earned high praise and the thanks of countless American servicemen.

Meanwhile Freud had sent Edward a note of thanks for the cigars and included a copy of his book, *The General Introduction to Psychoanalysis.* Bernays read it and took from it the idea that humans were fundamentally emotional and irrational creatures. And he immediately recognized that for anyone in public life it was pointless to appeal to masses rationally if you want them to support something.

At the time Bernays was in the "propaganda" business. He realized that Freud's ideas offered a way to manipulate the masses and he wanted to promote Freud's notions but he didn't want to use the word "propaganda" which had bad connotations. During the war people realized that propaganda was used to present or promote information that was misleading, dishonest or exploitative. So Bernays coined the term "public relations" for the same thing. He began to argue that the future of marketing, advertising and politics was to find ways of appealing to the emotional side of people through symbols and the language of metaphor. The aim was to get people to react in the way that you wanted, quickly. Bernays believed that in order for free market capitalism to flourish man's desires must overshadow needs. America had to be transformed from a mentality of "wanted" versus "needed". He showed American corporations how they could make people want things they didn't need by systematically linking mass-produced goods to their unconscious desires.

And corporations were willing to listen because they believed they had a huge problem. Mass production had become an efficient technology and was becoming bigger all the time. Top management of corporations was worried about overproduction; i.e. that people might actually stop buying things once they had what they needed. After all up until that time, the working classes only bought things that they needed. Bernays started to say: "I can connect with people emotionally and manipulate how they feel about themselves so they will buy whatever I make them unconsciously desire". The new creed was that you buy things to express your inner sense of self. Bernays could tap in to deepest desires and fears and use them for corporate purposes. The idea of democracy was changing the relations of power. The Bernays idea of democracy was changing the relations of power even if you stimulate an irrational self so that business can grow. The American citizen's importance to the country was changing from being a citizen to being a consumer. Intellectual journalists became fascinated and frightened. Prior to the 1920's the belief that human beings could be trusted to make rational decisions was a most fundamental principle to democracy. The Bernays pitch was that this fundamental principle was essentially wrong. Emotional desires could be stimulated, and then sated with consumer goods.

While Bernays was getting rich, Freud was on the verge of bankruptcy in the 1920's. Freud wrote to Bernays to ask if he could help. Bernays immediately sent Uncle Sigmund money but also he got Freud published in the United States. Bernays in effect became Freud's agent in America, using all the new tricks of PR. He made his uncle acceptable, promoted him and continued to cash in. And Bernays continued to generate good money for Freud in subsequent publications in the U.S. Though there were occasional difficulties between the two of them. For example, Bernays wanted Freud to write an article for Cosmopolitan Magazine on the place of the woman in the home. Freud refused because he thought that the idea was too vulgar. It is the view of the documentary film that without Bernays Freud may have been a more insignificant figure or at least not have had the influence that he did in becoming well known to the public. The documentary film's perspective is that it was public relations that made Freud so famous, more than it was academic credibility.

The "Century of the Self "documentary essentially says that from the 1920's onward people have become confused by Bernays and others with regard to the difference between individual needs and wants. For example one of Bernays' most notorious "successes" was to make it socially acceptable for women to smoke.

It was the president of the American Tobacco Company who recognized that an important part of his market was not being tapped, given that women did not smoke, at least in public. He hired Bernays to expand the sales of Lucky Strike cigarettes to women. Bernays applied his talent to the problem. Recognizing that women were still riding high on the suffrage movement, Bernays consulted Dr. A.A. Brill, a leading New York psychoanalyst, to find out the psychological basis for women's smoking. Brill said that cigarettes were equated subconsciously with penises, which women were envious of. He gave Bernays the idea that if he could connect cigarettes with the idea of challenging male power, smoking in public could be sold to women. So Bernays came up with an idea for presenting cigarettes as "torches of freedom". He proceeded to stage an event at the annual Easter Day Parade, held in New York and attracting thousands, to introduce this totally irrational notion to American womanhood. He got a group of rich debutantes to agree to hide cigarettes in their clothing and, at a given signal, light up together. Bernays informed the press ahead of time so that photographers were present in droves and stories appeared in newspapers throughout America.

Bernays's efforts had a lasting effect. He persuaded female film stars to smoke ostentatiously on screen, thus endorsing smoking cigarettes as respectable and desirable. Women began to smoke in millions because he had linked smoking to feelings of independence, power and freedom. This was one of several tricks of mass persuasion by using the practice of associative product placement in movies. And Bernays began the strategy of selling cars as symbols of male sexuality. The perspective of the film is that consumerism had an ideology, just as much as fascism or communism did. Consumerism became another way of managing the masses in an age of mass democracy. "People like Bernays were the first architects of that. The model they used was fundamentally the pessimistic Freudian view that we are emotional, irrational creatures. We live in that tent. We don't think outside it at the moment. That is what we are. According to the film the Freudian view denies another aspect of human nature, which is being able to think outside of yourself, to think about others, to think rationally." [6]

But Bernays came to some pushback against his approach after Roosevelt was elected in 1932. Roosevelt believed that humans could be rational. He rejected the ideas of Bernays. He argued that people could be trusted to know what they wanted. Roosevelt appealed to human dignity. He brought in the pollsters Gallup and Roper so that each week it could be reported what the nation was thinking, week to week. Roosevelt's aim was a collective awareness against the unfettered power of capitalism that had caused the financial crisis of the early 1930's. Government warned of the unscrupulous manipulation of the press by business. So after the 1936 election, and under the baton of Bernays, business launched a public relations campaign for an emotional connection between American citizens and Business. By 1939 Bernays produced a huge exhibit, on the order of a world's fair, that was a vision of a future world with the consumer as king. The exhibit was titled "Democricity". It was elaborate propaganda showing how human desires were read and fulfilled by business and the free market. "All would be me" so to speak, via the free market. The free market was something that was guided by peoples' will versus government. Bernays claim and his pitch to businesses was that this was a better form of democracy. Privately Bernays did not believe that democracy could ever work due to Freud's theories of primitive unconscious desires and feelings that overwhelmed rational thought. Bernays really believed that it was too dangerous to ever let the masses have control over their own lives. He believed that peoples' desires are in charge, not people. The Bernays solution was passive consumers in lieu of an active citizenry.

In Part 2 of the "Century of the Self", the perspective is about how Freud's ideas about the unconscious mind were used by those in power in post-war America. By that time politicians and planners had come to believe Freud's underlying premise, that deep within all human beings were dangerous and irrational desires and fears. They were convinced that it was the unleashing of these instincts that had led to the barbarism of Nazi Germany. Nazis were the anti-democratic gone wild. So, to stop it ever happening again, they set out to find ways to control this hidden enemy within the human mind. And it was Anna Freud, now the acknowledged leader of the psychoanalytic movement, along with her cousin Eddie Bernays, who provided the ideas that were used by the United States government, big business, and the CIA to develop techniques to manage and control the minds of the American people. But this was not a cynical exercise in manipulation. Those in power believed that the only way to make democracy work and create a stable society was to repress the savage barbarism that the psychoanalysts told them lurked just under the surface of normal American life.

What had happened was that during the war forty-nine percent of all soldiers evacuated from combat were found to be suffering severe mental health problems. In desperation the army turned to psychoanalysts. It was the first time such attention had been given to the feelings and anxieties of such a large number of ordinary people. The refugee psychoanalysts from Europe worked with American psychiatrists, using techniques developed by Freud to take the men back to their past. Analysts were convinced that the breakdowns were not the direct result of the fighting. They believed that the stress of combat had merely triggered old childhood memories of violent feelings and desires, which soldiers had repressed because they were too frightening. To the psychoanalysts this mass of traumatized soldiers was overwhelming proof of Freud's theory. Even though victory in the Second World War was celebrated as a triumphant reassertion of democracy, many policy makers were privately worried about the implications of the analysis of the soldiers. Policy makers believed that the complicity of so many ordinary Germans in mass killings during the war showed how easily irrational forces could break through and overwhelm democracy. And it was believed that there was "much more suffering in the post-war U.S. life than one would imagine from the advertisements of what the United States was supposed to be"[7] Psychoanalysts were convinced that they not only understood dangerous unconscious forces but that they knew how to control them too. They offered to use their techniques to create democratic individuals, because democracy, left to it-self, could not be relied upon to do this.

In 1946 President Truman signed the National Mental Health Act born directly out of the wartime "discoveries" by psychoanalysts. The Act recognized mental illness as a national problem. A vast project began in America to apply the ideas of psychoanalysis to the masses. Psychological guidance centers were set up in hundreds of towns staffed by psychiatrists who believed it was their job to control the hidden forces inside the minds of millions of ordinary Americans. Anna Freud's continued work was in large part the basis for so much mental health funding. People could learn to regulate their emotions in appropriate ways. Counselors were trained to apply psychoanalysis to marriage guidance. And social workers were sent out to visit peoples' homes and to advise on the psychological structure of family life.

This was only the beginning of the rise to power of psychoanalysis in America. Psychoanalysts moved into big business to use their techniques, not just to create model citizens, but model consumers. The Institute of Motivational Research was set up, to explore why people behave as they do, and buy as they do. And then psychoanalyst Ernest Dichter set up the first "focus group" to discover the hidden motivations of people, in connection with particular products. Corporations and advertising agencies all started rushing, then, to employ psychoanalysts. They called them "the depth boys". What happened was that a group of psychoanalysts took what Bernays had begun and invented a whole range of techniques to get inside and manage the unconscious mind of the consumer. By the early 1950's the ideas of psychoanalysis had penetrated deep into American life. The psychoanalysts themselves became rich and powerful and had many famous politicians, writers and show business celebrities as patients. And as their ideas took hold, a new elite began to emerge in politics, social planning, and the business world. What linked them was the assumption that the masses were fundamentally irrational. The way to manage a free market democracy, like America, was to use their psychological understanding to control this irrationality in the interests of everyone.

Then, after the Soviet Union exploded its first hydrogen bomb in 1953, fear of nuclear war and communism gripped the United States. The American government again turned to Eddie Bernays for help and he advised President Eisenhower that appeals to reason in the face of the communist threat were pointless. Instead, to win the Cold War, these mass fears should actually be encouraged and manipulated but in such a way that they could be used as a weapon against communism. For example, the United Fruit Company owned vast banana plantations in Guatemala and in effect controlled the country through pliable dictators. The company asked Bernays for help when a new *democratically elected* socialist was elected president and refused to play ball with United Fruit Company. Public Relations painted the new leader as a dangerous communist recruited by Moscow and news media were bombarded with "information" that Moscow intended to use Guatemala as a base to attack America; i.e. a Soviet outpost in our back yard. Eisenhower agreed to the Guatemalan leader being toppled in secret, and the American people saw it as a great triumph when the elected leader was forced to flee his country.

Part 3 of "Century of the Self" shows how, in the 1960's the influence of Freudian ideas in America was challenged by a group of psychotherapists who believed that the inner self did not need to be repressed and controlled. It could be encouraged to express itself. This happened because psychoanalysis fell out of favor. It became impossible to hide the fact that as a therapy it just didn't seem to work very well. Famous patients like Marilyn Monroe committed suicide. Anna Freud was also discredited, in part. One of the children that Anna had analyzed after the War was the daughter of Anna's close friend Dorothy Burlingham. The analysis had apparently been quite successful. But the girl actually came back from America as an adult and committed suicide in the Freud's London house where Anna still lived. There was also a famous experiment, funded by the CIA, in which the head of the American Psychiatric Association, Dr. Ewan Cameron, tried to remove the dangerous inner forces from mentally ill people. He bombarded them with drugs and ECT to erase their memories of the past and replace them with positive material, played to them on tape. All he ended up with was dozens of people with memory loss.

Such events marked the end of the political influence of psychoanalysis. At the same time, people on the political left in America became fed up with having, as they saw it, ideas implanted in their minds by big business and the state, a process directly stemming from Freudian ideas, particularly from Anna Freud and Eddie Bernays. *The Hidden Persuaders,* a powerful book by Vance Packard, accused psychoanalysts of reducing people to puppets by manipulating their desires. Students in the mid-1960s accused corporate America of brainwashing people in order to keep them docile, while the Viet Nam war was pursued. There was the Democratic Convention in 1968 Chicago where police turned on demonstrating students, and then the killing of students at Kent State University in 1969. In the face of such powerful assaultive opposition the Left fell apart as a political force. Individuals began to look for new ways to bring about change. They turned to the ideas of renegade psychoanalysts like Wilhelm Reich and Fritz Perls.

Even though Reich was dead by this time one of his students, Fritz Perls had set himself up as a psychotherapist guru in a rundown motel called Esalen at Big Sur, California. Perls developed a form of encounter group to push individuals to publicly express the feelings that society had told them were dangerous and should be repressed. Perls and his colleagues believed they were creating ways that allowed individuals to free their minds of social constraints. Out of this, they thought, would develop new autonomous beings independent of society.This proved to be an enormously attractive idea to millions. From the late sixties into the seventies, thousands flocked to Esalen. From being obscure and fringe, it quickly became the center of a national movement for personal transformation, the "me" generation. The movement was a disaster but nevertheless business realized that it could be exploited. It was in the interest of business to encourage people to feel they were unique individuals and then sell ways to them to express that individuality. Once again business turned to techniques developed by Freudian psychoanalysts to read the inner desires of people; i.e., focus groups. The whole thing took off when one entrepreneur, Werner Erhard who started "EST", claimed they could teach 200-odd people at a time to find out how to "be themselves" on weekend courses. There were similar programs, like Exegis, that were developed in Britain.

The core idea was that there was no fixed, innate self. This meant that you could be anything you wanted to be. Erhard truly believed that we are trapped by the idea that we have a self and that defusing the notion that you have a true self is empowering. What he didn't realize was that by doing that to people he also liberated big business because it meant that business could say: "you can have any identity you want, be whatever you want to be, and we will sell you whatever you need to express your identity." People who went to his courses came out incredibly greedy and materialist and exploiters of other people. Families were wrecked by it. It was extreme narcissism but a powerful idea that arguably led, in part, to the new self-expressive consumerism that rose in the 80's and dominated life in the 90's. Many "EST" graduates also went into management consulting.

Another example of the anti-Freudian movement was Maslow's idealistic notion of "self-actualization", which became a mantra in counseling and education circles. This is the idea that people can, if given enough "space", become completely self-directed and free of society. It has been called romanticism because it ignores the impact of life experiences on the brain, such as education stress, etc and how that affects who we become. But in essence it is still a Freudian idea, that fundamentally we have this emotional self. One example of the naivety of Maslow's movement was how easily and quickly it was exploited and used. Maslow's hierarchy of needs became the basis of what is now called lifestyle marketing, which is so powerful throughout the western world and underpins much of modern consumerism.

Part 4 of "Century of the Self", the final episode, is about political use of consumerism. It shows how the satisfaction of individual feelings and desires were seized upon by Left wing politicians in order to regain power in the 1990's.

Conservative politicians, especially those who believed in the free market, have a pessimistic view of human beings anyway, so they picked up on it easily. Ronald Reagan was elected on the slogan of "let the people rule" Margaret Thatcher flourished on the idea of giving people what they wanted through the free market. Both Reagan and Thatcher encouraged business to take over the role of fulfilling people's desires. But politicians who had grown up in the postwar era with the belief that the state should be run by a paternalistic elite who could rationally imagine what people needed, inspire and lead them, were late in "getting it". This was the case even though the economic crisis of the 1970's showed that the paternalistic way had apparently failed. By the early 1990's the Left were faced with the problem that their electorate, as Clinton's advisors said to him, thought of themselves as consumers.

In the early 90's in Britain a political strategist, Philip Gould commissioned focus groups to find out the electorate's underlying feelings. On the basis of his findings he tried to persuade Labor to make concessions to the aspiration class. The Shadow Chancellor in Britain, at the time, refused to have anything to do with such ideas and insisted Labor, if elected, would put up taxes to fund public services. Gould's ideas continued to be rejected by Labor so Gould went to join Clinton's campaign in America. Clinton bought the idea that people didn't want to pay raised taxes to fund benefits for wider society but he couldn't honor promises not to raise taxes because the financial implications turned out to be too huge. At the start of his administration Clinton tried to talk about real ideals; such as homeless, poor, schools, medical care, etc. But the middle class felt betrayed. Clinton started losing support and, in desperation, took the advice that he would have to turn politics into a form of consumer business—identifying and meeting inner desires. So all the Democratic traditional policies were dropped and he concentrated on meeting the concerns of swing voters.

The ploy was a great success! It was short-term policies that had no vision. And it started happening in Britain too. When Tony Blair became leader of New Labor in 1994, Gould was his strategy adviser. He ran almost nightly focus groups, again concentrating on the swinging voters and the issues that mattered to them. When Blair was first in office, he didn't pay much attention to the railways because focus groups hadn't identified them as a high priority. But as soon as the rail crashes started happening, everyone blamed New Labor for not putting more money into the railways. They couldn't have, of course, because they had no long-term strategy—just what mattered in the short term, to win the voters.

Politicians had a complete failure of imagination and of nerve, particularly in Britain and America. They had nothing to offer so they turned to focus groups and consumer techniques, perhaps with a sense of blessed relief. In effect they said "We haven't got any ideas so let's ask people what they want and give it to them". And then they became trapped with no room for maneuvers. Their policies became increasingly dictated by short-termism and selfishness, in other words: consumerism. Policies are decided in committees that are inhibited by reports from focus groups. And these decisions are always biased by urges to gain political advantage and please the people. This means that no government can ever be in tune with reality.

It seems that consumerism is a way of managing human beings as much as it is a way of selling them things. The roots of it lie very explicitly back in the 1920's. We have forgotten this but it grew out of Bernays' ideological idea about managing the masses at a time when democracy was emerging. Back then governments argued about controlling in a totalitarian way, fascist or communist. But another way to control people, in the name of Democracy, was found through consumerism. Consumerism is an ideological response to the need government has to control the masses, and it is a very successful way of managing people. The consumer democracy that was embraced in the U.S. and by Labor in Britain has faced them with a dilemma. The system of consumer democracy has trapped them into a series of short-term and often contradictory policies. As more things go wrong there are increasing demands that they face from constituents who (now) want a grander vision. Electorates expect leaders to use the power of government to deal with problems of growing inequality and the decaying social fabric of the country. But to do this, they will have to appeal to the electorate to think outside of their own individual self-interest. We have forgotten that we can be more than that; that there are other sides to human nature. And now, although we feel we are free, in reality we, like the politicians, have become the slaves of our own desires.[8] It will take some historical crisis to come along, like a war or "something" but "some crisis" *will change everything.*[9] Public Relations people believe that consumerism fed by focus groups is a new and much better form of democracy. What the "Century of the Self" four-part documentary argues is that this is a very limited idea of democracy. But that the old paternalistic idea isn't right either. That is why the documentary film is left open-ended. And that is why the remainder of this Foreword to Symposium 2009 will attempt to begin an open-ended conversation with Psychoanalysis so that we may develop an integrated, potentially multi-faceted relationship within the future of a democratic society.

Beginning A Conversation

The history that is depicted above is the documentary film producer's point-of-view. But the fact of Eddie Bernays is real. The personal relationship between Eddie Bernays and Freud has been explored in other literature and the reader may pursue other sources as they are of interest[10] Biographer Larry Tye in *The Father of Spin* says "Anyone who knew Eddie Bernays knew how much he took from his illustrious uncle, Sigmund Freud. But few knew how much he gave back". "Eddie recognized the value of Freud's papers, monetarily and historically, to his uncle and to himself. In the end, however, Eddie was preoccupied with the public arena while matters private and inward looking captivated Freud. Eddie was, in essence, a sociologist while Freud remained a committed psychologist. But while Freud sought to liberate people from their subconscious drives and desires, Eddie sought to exploit those passions."[11]

An article written about Bernays in the 1930's praised him: "Only poets delude themselves with the notion that love, that is to say sex, causes the world to revolve. Mr. Bernays knows that it is really money that furnishes the motive power. The mass psychologist moreover goes further than the psychoanalyst who can do no more than explain what has already taken place. Eddie can foretell the future. . . . *His* science, once understood, is really very simple. What he does is to create a demand by molding the public mind" (Henry Pringle, "The Mass Psychologist," in the *American Mercury,* 1930).

Then, two years later: "Bernays is a philosopher, not a mere businessman. He is a nephew of that other great philosopher, Dr. Sigmund Freud. Unlike his distinguished uncle, he is not known as a practicing psychoanalyst, but he is a psychoanalyst just the same, for he deals with the science of unconscious mental processes. His business is to treat unconscious mental acts by conscious ones. The great Viennese doctor is interested in releasing the pent-up libido of the individual; his American nephew is engaged in releasing and directing the suppressed desires of the crowd". (By John T. Flynn, "The Science of Ballyhoo" in *Atlantic Monthly,* 1932)

But there was also severe criticism of Bernays's methods, especially a decade later in the 1940s. Reviewing Bernays's book *Take Your Place at the Peace Table,* 1945, the reviewer wrote: (The book) is a mixture of honest liberalism and incipient cynical fascism. There is much talk of the individual common man and open discussion and truth and accuracy, but much more of molding public opinion by various tools and weapons and plans and strategies." "The author presumably intends only welfare and happiness for humanity, but his methods are largely identical with those portrayed in Chapters VI and XI of *Mein Kampf"* (Pitman B. Potter, *The American Political Science Review,* 1945)

Writing forty-two years later, author Marvin Olasky says that Pitman Potter missed the point. Such a blending of liberalism and fascism, Olasky says, "was exactly what Bernays believed to be essential, given his understanding of the failure of nineteenth-century liberalism, and the twentieth-century 'necessity' of uniting liberalism with social control to avoid chaos." As for Bernays's endorsement of propaganda, Olasky adds, "if Hitler had hit upon the techniques and used them for evil purposes, then that would be all the more reason for liberals such as Bernays to use them before fascists had the chance." Olasky adds that it is inevitable that these techniques would be put into use and that man would not have the ability to resist them. Olasky writes, "Bernays believed we must be manipulative in order to save democracy. He believed that we have to burn the village in order to save it" (Marvin Olasky in *Corporate PublicRelations: A New Historical Perspective,* 1987).

Over the years Bernays found it hard to make his actions believable as consistent with his words. In 1986 when he wrote *The Later Years: Public Relations Insights* he tried to explain himself. He said of his very first book, *Crystallizing Public Opinion,* published in 1923: "I tried to lay down the principles, practices, and ethics of a new profession. I was unaware then that words, unless defined by law, are in the public domain and have the stability of soap bubbles." As biographer Larry Tye asks: How must Bernays have felt, when he learned in 1933 that Nazi propaganda chief Joseph Goebbels was using *Crystallizing Public Opinion* as a basis for his destructive campaign against the Jews of Germany? "Bernays heard about it from Karl von Wiegand, foreign correspondent for the Hearst papers, who had visited with Goebbels in Germany and been given a tour of the Goebbels library. While scholars still debate the extent to which the Nazis used Bernays's works, Goebbels did employ techniques nearly identical to those used by Bernays, skillfully exploiting symbols by making Jews into scapegoats and Hitler into the embodiment of righteousness; manipulating the media by trumpeting Nazi triumphs on the battlefield and hiding their extermination campaigns; and vesting unheard-of power in state propagandists just as Bernays had advised in *Crystallizing.*"

Bernays was savvy enough never to retell the Goebbels tale in the 1930's and 1940's, when it could have tarnished his image. But he couldn't resist recounting von Wiegand's story in his autobiography, published in 1965. News that his book was on Goebbels's shelf "shocked me," Bernays wrote. "But I knew any human activity can be used for social purposes or misused for antisocial ones. Obviously the attack on the Jews of Germany was no emotional outburst of the Nazis, but a deliberate, planned campaign." Nevertheless, (very) deep down, Bernays had prior experience with what he had unleashed. As early as 1932 he orchestrated a campaign on behalf of a national commission that was proposing group medical practices, group payment through private and public insurers, and more emphasis on training midwives and nursing attendants. Bernays was determined that the commission's good work be recognized, so he convened hearings across the country, encouraged newspapers to print stories with local angles on the national themes, mailed thousands of letters and spoke on radio shows. But Bernays was outmaneuvered by the American Medical Association, which borrowed Bernays's own tactics to convince the public that the commission's proposals were dangerous. "The alignment is clear", argued a two-and-a-half-page AMA editorial. "On the one side the forces representing the great foundations, public health officialdom, social theory—even Socialism and Communism—inciting to revolution; on the other side, the organized medical profession of this country urging an evolution guided by controlled experimentation which will observe the principles that have been found through the centuries to be necessary to the sound practice of medicine." Being beaten at his own game was so unsettling that Bernays was still steaming forty-five years later. "As a result of this effort", he told an interviewer, the AMA "was able to stop medical progress in this country until President Lyndon Johnson came along some thirty years after."

So now let those of us who read this Volume and remember the event of Symposium, 2009, think about an irony that has been around psychoanalysis, in an unspoken way, for far too long. It seems to be a more salient irony given that Freud's particular genius was in his resolution of polarities that torment the soul. That good and evil grow from a common root.

But the existence of the relationship between these two, a history that has always been around psychoanalysis, though not "of" psychoanalysis, may give us a clue to an inherent irony in Symposium 2009 and within Psychoanalysis. Isn't it ironic that the particular topics of our Symposium were all fostered, nurtured and manipulated by Eddie Bernays and the professional industry that he himself founded, almost a century ago? Bernays did it with "psychoanalysis"! His profession is only getting better at it and they do it, in the name of democracy and freedom, with techniques that came from psychoanalysis. More specifically, they do it with techniques that have perverted Freud's intentions for human understanding. The story of Bernays could (should?) have been a paper at *Symposium 2009*! So is there something not only ironic but also uncanny about the story of Bernays? And can we use it in our ongoing conversation as a way to work through psychoanalysis in order to relocate the possibilities for psychoanalysis within the future of a free society?

What the story of Bernays has caused me to wonder is whether its eerie history represents an unconscious presence that sustains *The Prisonhouse*, as Arnold Goldberg described it, two decades ago. In the first half of the 20th century, psychoanalysis was poised for a great era ahead. We went in to decline as psychoanalytic science and treatment efficiency were questioned. Psychiatry removed us from a position of power. We haven't been able to get ourselves up and running again in an empowering way. Yet all the while a most perverse and limited use of psychoanalytic truth has flourished.

During these decades of decline we have retreated to our independent psychoanalytic institutes where we talk to each other and teach the competing psychoanalytic theories. We keep repeating ourselves, as we were. It is as if we live, literally, in the State of Developmental Arrest. Can the portal that was opened at *Symposium 2009* give us an opportunity for our own therapeutic action? Is it possible that we both know and don't know that there is knowledge within us that must be brought forward to make of ourselves a truly human professional life? [12]

Perhaps the time has come for psychoanalysis to enact a renewed version of its particular genius, the resolution of polarities, once again. Our renewed version of the genius that is psychoanalysis should be appropriate for these times. The renewal of psychoanalysis (*not of Freud*)[13] in the 21st century should essentially be the recognition that our profession needs to bring a resolution to the polarities that remain within us. How do we mobilize the reality that resolution of ourselves must become a lifetime professional task, going forward? "The Price of Freedom is Eternal Vigilance."[14]

In Eric Kandel's recent autobiography[15] he describes an invitation he received at the time that he received the Nobel Prize. The invitation was from the President of Austria who wanted to honor Kandel as a Nobel Laureate of Viennese origin. Kandel took the opportunity to suggest a symposium entitled "Austria's Response to National Socialism: Implications for Scientific and Humanistic Scholarship." Kandel says that his purpose was to compare Austria's response to the Hitler period, which was one of denial of any wrongdoing, with Germany's response, which was to try to deal honestly with the past.

Suppose we frame *Symposium 2009,* within our own minds as follows: It was an extremely productive "session" that came to an end when the analyst informed us "unfortunately 'our time is up' for today". Since then we have had time to experience some working through process from the content of the Symposium. Given the background story of the reality of Eddie Bernays, and the publication of this Volume, how might we envision a future Symposium(s)? As corollary to Kandel's example, suppose we prepared the following:

"A Psychoanalytic Outreach to Philosophy, Biology and to Economics: Implications for Scientific and Humanistic Scholarship."

My purpose here is this: Psychoanalysis has been living for decades, now, as if the truth that it holds is an undervalued asset. The more important reality is that Eddie Bernays'simplistic manipulation of the asset was, in human terms, as overvalued as credit default swaps on low-income mortgages. Nevertheless, we participated.

Psychoanalysis was young when Bernays came along. There hadn't been time yet for our own psychological structure to deepen in a way that could handle the ever-deepening and unpredictable complexities of what we had begun. But psychoanalysis has got to find a way to change the fundamental perception with which it is seen by the likes of Biology and Economics. This can only come from ourselves changing our own fundamental perception about us. Have we been responding to our guilt by denying any wrongdoing? More importantly can psychoanalysis try to deal honestly with our past? If psychoanalysis can enact a stage of developmental maturity for open discussion of ourselves perhaps we will be able to laugh at ourselves as we remember (some) of the times from when we were younger.We have to evolve our maturity enough to get the ironic joke about ourselves within the backdrop of our past. For example: Did you hear about the psychoanalysts who once thought they could control democracy and capitalism? Hah! And when we are able to "get the joke" we will be free of the *Prisonhouse,* more flexible and able to integrate with other disciplines that will help psychoanalysis to deepen itself. We will enhance our own psychological structure to withstand change and to sustain growth in unpredictable ways.

When you read the extraordinary papers that are contained in this Volume, think about how the analysis of our profession might unfold, given the productivity of the session that was Symposium 2009. If humanities and the sciences can be unified, how does psychoanalysis roll up its sleeves, join the interdisciplinary research team, and help to engineer the unification bridge? The complex distal vision for humanity has always belonged to us. Eddie Bernays never got it. Or if he "got it" perhaps Bernays knew that he could not *live* it. For all of the communication between him and his uncle perhaps neither one could move to bring forward what each must have known and not known about himself and about the other. Can we be anything other than empathic to each of them and henceforth more empathic to ourselves as we struggle for our unique place and a unique voice within the future?

END NOTES

1. "When Socrates asks, 'What is involved in becoming truly human?' he is asking what would be the highest development of ourselves, what is the most noble and fine in becoming a human being, and how can we in the deepest sense become ourselves? Socrates recognizes that living with these questions—genuinely living with these questions as continually renewed questions—is a lifetime task." "It is of the essence of Socratic irony that the question is a genuine question". From Jonathan Lear: *Therapeutic Action (An Earnest Plea for Irony),* 2003, p.75.

2. See Eric Kandel, "Biology and the Future of Psychoanalysis: A New Intellectual Framework for Psychiatry Revisited", originally published in the *American Journal of Psychiatry,* Volume 156, Number 4, 1999, pages 505–524. The paper is reprinted in Kandel, Eric: *Psychiatry, Psychoanalysis, and the New Biology of Mind*, 2005, American Psychiatric Publishing.

3. Arnold Goldberg: *Prisonhouse of Psychoanalysis*. 1990

4. See Jonathan Lear: *Love and Its Place in Nature,* (1990), especially Chapter 7 on "Radical Evaluation"

5. The history that is described here comes mainly from the documentary film footage, "Century of the Self" which is available free, online, and also from an extensive interview with the film's producer, Adam Curtis, which first appeared in the *Human Givens Journal,* Volume 9, No.3, 2002. "Human Givens Institute" is an organization in the UK that offers professional education in mental health and also education for the public and organizations. The Human Givens Institute approach is described as one that is bio-psycho-social.

   In a limited way, for some background depth of understanding Edward Bernays relationship with Freud, I used a fine autobiography of Bernays titled: *The Father of Spin* by journalist Larry Tye, 1998, Crown Publishers, New York.

6. This is a direct quote from Adam Curtis, the "Century of Self "film producer, in the published interview with him, 2002, *Human Givens Journal.*

7. This comes from psychoanalyst Martin Bergmann, interview footage from the documentary. Bergmann was one of the psychoanalyst refugees from Europe. Little did he know perhaps that what he was seeing of advertised America was there due to the professional public relations skills of Bernays, nephew to Sigmund Freud?

8. Is there an uncanny corollary here to Goldberg's *Prisonhouse of Psychoanalysis*?

9. This remark is from the published interview with Adam Curtis, 2002. Symposium 2009 was produced after "the crisis" that did come along and changed everything; the financial crisis.

10. Elisabeth Young-Bruehl's biography of *Anna Freud;* Edward Bernays own Autobiography, the Library of Congress Letters between Bernays and Freud that were exchanged 1919–1933, Larry Tye's biography *The Father of Spin*. Other sources are surely available via Freud scholars.

11. Tye in *Father of Spin,* page 197.

12. See Jonathan Lear's *Therapeutic Action (An Earnest Plea for Irony),* Chapter 2.

13. Nor of other theoretical heroes.

14. John Maynard Keynes quoted in "Freedom" by Donald W. Winnicott, in *Home is Where We Start From.*

15. Kandel: *The Emergence of a New Science of Mind,* 2006.

Leslie Shaw, Ph.D.
980 North Michigan (#1400)
Chicago, IL 60611
Leslie@leslieshaw.com

Ken Winarick

INTRODUCTION

It seems that greed is everywhere, not that it hasn't always been, but now it has taken on new dimensions. *The New York Times* has described it as an "engrossing orgy of greed, graft, cronyism, and corruption" (Stanley 2008), scandals that both excite and appall us. This orgy, however, doesn't have much to do with sexuality, as it is typically understood. When "greed trumps lust" and love is lost, sadistic pleasure prevails.

We are drawn into a world of ruthless aggression, in which the accumulation of wealth and power take precedence over all other considerations. People are treated as part objects to be exploited, damaged, and controlled. Even the fleeting recognition of otherness is avoided at all costs, making mature moral responsibility all but impossible. The consequences have been a far reaching economic and social calamity that touches us all. The damage to the individual and society, however, goes beyond the actual financial losses, which have been substantial. to the often devastating subjective meanings of the losses for the individual. It also includes the destructive influence of the highly visible, financially successful but morally corrosive subcultures that stimulate greed and envy and infuse sibling and oedipal competition with even greater aggression and fear.

How do psychoanalysts understand this? And what, if any, remedy does psychoanalysis have to offer? Is it just that we need more regulation in the form of new laws and/or more regulators to buttress internal controls that seem so easily overwhelmed? Or are the determinants more complex and tenacious and the solution more difficult? If it is the latter, and I believe it is, psychoanalysis has much to offer. Psychoanalysis offers us a dynamic understanding of personality that takes into account aspects of the mind that are unconscious but exert a powerful force driving the unbridled greed that is so destructive to the victims and, ultimately, to the victimizers.

This symposium explores greed in different forms: in the pursuit of money, of sex, of power, and particularly of political power. To the extent that greed infuses these strivings, it should be no surprise then that all three are often strivings actively pursued by the same individual.

In some instances one of the strivings may initially predominate. Once it loses meaning, either through success or disappointment, a shift to another often occurs. For example a greedy striving for money, if successful, is often replaced by a striving for political power.

What underlies this commonality and what are its defining characteristics? The answer I believe requires a journey into Klein's theory of mind. Klein's theory is a journey into an inner world of unconscious fantasies of destruction and persecution, of omnipotent fantasies and beliefs buttressed by primitive defenses. It is a journey into an inner world of blurred boundaries between self and others and, consequently, a profound alienation from one's true self. Klein (1957) believed greed developed from the earliest experiences of being fed or not fed, of having hunger frustrated or gratified. Klein inferred that fantasies, fears, and mental processes occurred in the minds of infants as a consequence of these early oral experiences. The possibility of verifying these inferences in any substantive way has been justifiably questioned. Even so, this does not invalidate the usefulness and relevance of the dynamic constellation of unconscious fantasies and defenses that Klein postulated for understanding the current functioning of those consumed by pathological greed. The developmental link between greed and frustrating or gratifying oral experiences cited by both Abraham (1924) and Klein (1957) should not be dismissed or ignored. There is an intuitive relationship between greed and hunger that has always been part of our lexicon and is part of the standard definition of greed.

It is worthwhile to review the unconscious fantasies, defensive maneuvers, and mental processes that Klein described. as they illustrate important aspects of adult mental functioning. They appear to resonate closely with the pathology of the psychopathic personalities we read about daily. To borrow a phrase from Horney, (1937) they are driven by the " pursuit of power, prestige, and possession."

To Klein, recurrent early oral experiences of frustration and gratification are powerful stimuli both for loving and for destructive hating feelings. These, with too much privation and deprivation, intensify aggression and diminish love. Aggression then becomes dominant. It is transformed into greed and greedy fantasies of biting, tearing, devouring, scooping out and annihilating the frustrating source of insufficient food, the bad breast. Furthermore, greed stimulates envy of the giver who has the food and control. So that whatever is given becomes, in fantasy, something that is sadistically taken, the value of which must be denigrated as an act of vengeance against the envied object. The consequence is a vicious circle of deprivation and frustration and a sense of never having enough, which leads to a further intensification of greedy sadistic fantasies. These fantasies are then projected, distorting the image of the hated, depriving object. Thus, generating a fear that the object, now filled with greedy and destructive fantasies, will attack and devour in return.

These fantasies result in what Klein has described as persecutory anxiety; a paranoid fantasy, sustained and intensified by projection and introjection that mobilizes primitive defenses. These split the images of the good and bad objects in order to preserve the idealization of the good object and protect it from attacks from the bad object. Omnipotent fantasies are transformed into beliefs of unlimited power that develop to defend against persecutory anxiety. These omnipotent beliefs interact with projective identification to control or annihilate projected persecutory objects and to expel hated and devalued aspects of self. The ability to recognize a whole object, a person who is not a thing, requires that both loving and hating feelings can be experienced and tolerated toward the same person, one who is experienced as separate from the self with his/her own needs, wishes, vulnerability and pain. This recognition implies a tolerance for ambivalence which can be extremely difficult for someone who needs to split object representations and enact omnipotent fantasies of power and control with destructive exploitive attacks on others. However, if reality testing is not psychotically impaired, there must be some recognition, on an unconscious level, of the damage done to others. This recognition engenders unbearable guilt and depression. Thus, it becomes necessary to defend against it by denial of the damage done, by manic defenses that idealize strength, power and greed, and by a regressive retreat away from the painful implications of recognizing separateness, mutuality and interdependence. Ironically what appears on the surface as strength and independence, as being self-sufficient and not needing anybody, masks a compulsive sadistic dependence on others. Those others have the vital supplies that must be extracted and stolen continuously to bolster omnipotent fantasies and to satisfy wishes made insatiable by vicious circles of envy and greed. A controlling tie to others must be maintained to protect against attacks from those who in reality may have the power to hurt or harm but who are now filled with projective persecutory intent that makes them all the more dangerous. Perhaps the most tragic consequence is the loss of the ability to develop genuine intimacy and mature love. As Michael Balint (1952) has pointed out, this is an achievement that requires recognition of the separateness and wholeness of the other and tolerance of the frustration and depression associated with the inevitable limitations separateness imposes.

Betty Joseph (1960) in a prescient article fifty years ago, described the psychodynamics and, particularly, the relationship between greed and envy and the omnipotent defenses of a psychopathic patient. Joseph described three interrelated characteristics that she believed were fundamental to the psychopath; first, "... the striking inability to tolerate any tension, second, a particular attitude towards objects and third, a specific combination of defenses... " Her patient could not tolerate inner conflict and anxiety. He was extremely demanding and controlling, greedy and exploitive and cruel towards others with no apparent concern. Because of his intense envy, he had to "spoil and waste" what he was able get. This resulted in more frustration and greed, illustrating the vicious circle described earlier.

The patient incorporated and magically identified with "idealized, successful and desirable figures" that allowed him to avoid depressive feelings and any sense of loss resulting from genuine dependency and attachment . Furthermore, since he imagined he possessed the powers and capacities of the idealized objects, he had to split off and project his "failed and wasted," devalued and despised aspects into others and attack them with ". . . violent accusations . . ." Similarly he would project his persecutory, harsh punitive super-ego into authority figures and then constantly struggle to evade and control them. At other times he would have to placate his inner persecutors, his inner judges, with bribes, rationalizations, and denials to prove that ". . . his criminal impulses were not as they seem. . . ." His unconscious guilt and his need to be punished, however, were never absent. They often resulted in getting arrested and punished for petty things to avoid more extreme punishment, guilt and depression. He projected his criminal impulses into others and vicariously identified with them thus being able to avoid more serious crimes. In this regard, he differed from those criminals about whom we read in the media who have been arrested and charged with serious criminal actions. The financial crimes with which they are charged may seem to them petty or of less significance than the unconscious, intensely envious and hateful destructive wishes from which they emanated.

These traits capture the essential elements of the character and unconscious fantasies and defenses of psychopathic personalities. Some seem to compartmentalize their psychopathy and maintain splits in their internal and external world that allow for more mature levels of functioning in some areas. With others it seems to take over their entire being. Bernie Madoff is an example of the latter; his greed and psychopathy is so extreme and pervasive that he serves as a good clinical example, as does the fictional Gordon Gekko played by Michael Douglas in the movie *Wall Street*. They present differently; Madoff has been described as affable and charismatic in some situations but more consistently reclusive, standoffish and aloof. Gekko is brash, arrogant, and narcissistically expansive. The underlying dynamics are much the same; the variation in behavior is accounted for by different defensive and expressive modes of character organization. Madoff has been the subject of extensive investigative reporting by *The New York Times*. Friends, elementary and high school acquaintances, investors and employees have been interviewed as well as an ex FBI expert on criminal behavior, and a forensic psychologist, both of whom described Madoff as fitting the description of a psychopathic personality with the now all too familiar traits of lying, grandiosity, and callousness toward others. These descriptions of Madoff, however, focus largely on the external, on the observable, and although they provide glimpses into his internal world they are limited in their vision of the core unconscious process operating, a vision that psychoanalysis is best equipped to provide.

Unfortunately I know little about Madoff's early upbringing, the nature and quality of his relationship to his parents, or of the formative influences in his life. Interviews with him and descriptions of him, however, provide important clues to the unconscious fantasies and defenses that seem to be central to to understanding him. Of particular interest is how the experts compared ". . . the world of white collar finance criminals to the world of serial criminals . . . " More specifically, Madoff was compared to the serial killer Ted Bundy. "Whereas Ted Bundy murdered people, Mr. Madoff murdered people's wallets, their bank accounts and their sense of financial security."

"Serial killers have control over the life and death of people . . . They played God and took their actual lives. . . . Madoff played God because he had control of people's finances and as a result, the life and death of their financial security by taking their money." These experts sensed the presence of primitive murderous unconscious fantasies that were transformed and enacted by stealing money and thus undermining his victims sense of security and safety. In Madoff's mind, this was the subjective equivalent of hurting, damaging and annihilating them, making them feel the intolerable insecurity and terror he tried so hard to defend against.

The experts also highlighted his grandiosity, his sense of entitlement, and his almost psychotic identification with Godlike powers of control over others and the belief that he was special and above the law.

These observations resonate with Klein's understanding of the nature and functions of grandiosity as a set of omnipotent fantasies that serve to defend against persecutory anxiety These factores render the world into a jungle where one is either predator or prey, or in the everyday parlance of Wall Street, one either eats what one kills or is killed by being eaten. . . . It is the world that Madoff and others like him inhabit and with which they cope by becoming, in fantasy and in actuality, powerful predators who protect themselves from attack by attacking and devouring others. They, as prey, are objectified and treated as thing-like containers, that must be looted and destroyed. Madoff's callousness and cruelty to others is by now well known. One wonders if there is any goodness in his life, any compartmentalized relationships where he can experience the whole, separate humaneness of another and a semblance of mature love. His relationship with his wife, and perhaps his sons, seems at first glance to offer this possibility. He has been married for almost fifty years to a woman who has consistently been described as sweet and lovely. They were reported to be inseparable, working together, traveling together, and dining together. The very model of a devoted wife and husband. Certainly questions were raised about how much she knew. If she knew and was complicit, then she had more in common with him than then was apparent, the two of them forming a psychopathic folie a deux. If not, then she was manipulated, lied to and victimized, like everyone else. If the latter is true, the closeness of their relationship makes his treatment of her all the more vicious. Madoff actively solicited investments from her close friends and their relatives, friends that she had known for years, some of the relationships dating as far back as high school.

Madoff also actively pursued relationships with Wall Street regulators, eventually becoming a trusted advisor who assisted in writing the regulations that applied to his business. Perhaps this allowed him to project his internal persecutory objects into the regulators and protect himself from their realistic and fantasized destructive attacks. His harsh punitive internal objects were then deposited outside himself in the regulators. Thus, it made the previously internal objects, now externalized, less frightening and more susceptible to manipulation and control than the destructive retaliatory objects of his internal world. Then, at least, on a conscious level, he was free of internal punishment and moral inhibition, and could pursue unfettered a ruthless agenda to annihilate and kill those he feared would do the same to him.

Not surprisingly, he now finds himself the object of the very thing he imagined in fantasy and feared most, murderous death threats from those he murdered financially. An enactment is co-created. His persecutors, now identified with his projected murderous rage, threaten him with death but he is protected by bodyguards and wears a bulletproof vest, behavior which he can now justify. Again, the danger is externalized, managed and controlled and made less frightening and more concrete than the fantasized dangers of his internal world.

One wonders about whether he has any sense of guilt and or any awareness of the pain and suffering he has caused others. Are there moments when he is able to sustain a differentiated sense of self and other and glimpse the damage he has done? Can he experience some remorse or need for reparation, or are his self-accusations and guilt so primitive and pervasive that he has to repress and defend against any recognition of responsibility? And finally, does being caught and confessing to his sons satisfy a guilty need to be punished or is it just the result of reality intruding on an unsustainable omnipotent fantasy? We can only speculate here from very limited data. If we had him in analysis we might be better able to answer these questions, although there is not much likelihood of that happening.

I turn now to a fictional character, Gordon Gekko, the Wall Street trader and raider in the movie *Wall Street* (1987), as a further illustration of a psychopathic personality whose internal world, at least as it is portrayed in the movie, is strikingly similar to Madoff's. Gordon Gekko is a fictional character brought to life by an actor, his psychopathic personality traits stand out in a dramatic, highly visible way that may not be representative of the more complex, conflictual inner world of a real person. As such, he cannot serve as a clinical example but rather his character as it is portrayed in the movie can serve to delineate and clarify some of the central dynamics operating in a psychopathic personality in which greed stands out as a central organizing force.

Gekko is ruthless and "... takes no prisoners ...," a direct quote from the movie. His greed, unlike Madoff's, is not hidden by an aloof, persona, but stands out in vivid relief as part of what Horney (1950) called his pride system. He openly brags about his conquests, takes obvious sadistic pleasure from defeating and hurting his rivals, and idealizes his greed, trumpeting its value while disdaining those who inhibit or hide their greed. Gekko's murderous fantasies are close to the surface and readily observable. When he feels he is close to completing a deal, he says to his traders "we are in the kill zone, lock and load." He refers to his best trader as "the terminator" and instructs him to "blow them away." He wants to see things flowing red, as in blood. He refers to brokers who can't beat the S & P 500 as "sheep who get slaughtered" and he refers to his young protégé, Bud Fox, as a member of "his gang." He has a handgun collection and shows his rival the gun of which he is most proud, a rare German Luger, just before he is about to damage him financially.

He projects and introjects his greedy murderous fantasies and experiences the world as a war zone in which he is constantly in danger of attack and persecution. He quotes *The Art of War,* a Chinese treatise on military strategy written in the sixth century, B.C. (Sun-Tzu, Cleary translation, 1988), to justify his illegal actions, and tells Bud that "it's trench warfare out there," implying that it's either kill or be killed, annihilate or be annihilated, or, on the most primitive level, eat or be eaten. In such a terrifying world the power to extract endless supplies of money and maintain control over others provides a precarious island of safety and an outlet for gratifying destructive wishes. Feelings for others and love have no place in this world of primitive oral aggression. In a moment of self-revelation, Gekko alludes to his feelings of inferiority and envy, due among other things to his public college baclground. Now he has gotten the best of "Ivy League schmucks who suck my kneecaps," an obvious displacement downward. He says he doesn't want Harvard MBAs working for him. He wants people who are "poor, smart and hungry" with "no feelings."

"If you need a friend, get a dog." He tells his ex-lover, "don't buy into the oldest myth, love. It was created by people to keep them from jumping out the window." To him people are part objects to be used and manipulated. He has affairs without any thought of the damage they could do to his wife. He "gives" his ex-lover to Bud in order to enable her to seduce and control him. In the end, he callously attempts to destroy

Bud's emerging goodness, the love he feels for his father, and his regret at having hurt and humiliated him.

The reciprocal relationship between greed and envy is most clearly seen through the eyes of Bud, a young, relatively poor stockbroker from a working-class background whose greed is constantly being stimulated and intensified by his envy of Gekko. He is envious of Gecko's wealth and power, his impressive home, extensive art collection, corporate jet, the beautiful women he can have at any time, and his seemingly unlimited ability to accumulate wealth and defeat and humiliate his rivals. Gekko flaunts his money, showing Bud a check for a million dollars, the money he made in one day, and gives it to Bud to invest for him. Bud is excited, thinking it is the opportunity he has always desperately wanted. But it's also a tease. It's like dangling food in front of a starving person and saying: it's mine and you can't have it. All you can do is to touch it and handle it and make it grow into more for me. Gekko tempts Bud with the possibility that he might get some for himself, but even if Bud does get more it can only provide temporary satisfaction. Gekko will always have more, and once the envied supplies are obtained they must be devalued and spoiled, belittled or lost. It is Gekko's attempt to extract revenge on the envied, withholding object and minimize the envy that will all too soon reappear. So there is never enough, the hunger never disappears It is insatiable, made all the more so by the need to sustain defensive omnipotent fantasies that depend on accumulating more and more.

This all comes together in the most memorable moment in the movie—the greed-is-good speech. Gekko makes it at a stockholders' meeting of a company he is planning to take over.

Here, Gekko justifies his attempt to take control of the company by viciously attacking the executives on the board of the company whose money and power he envies and wants to take for himself. He projects his aggressive greedy wishes into the executives whom he now perceives as enemies out to hurt him. As the largest shareholder, he sees them greedily stealing his money, rewarding themselves with high salaries and many perks, without doing anything of value for the company By getting control of the company he protects himself from their greedy attacks on his assets and manages to get their assets for himself. He disparages the executives, sarcastically stating that the law of evolution that holds in corporate America is survival of the unfittest, while in his book its either do it right or get eliminated. He splits off the bad, despised aspects of self, his sense of weakness and inferiority and projects them into the incompetent executives while aggrandizing his own power and strength. His devaluation of the executives also serves to de-humanize them, to turn them into bad part objects so that the depression and guilt associated with any recognition of the hurt and damage done to them can be avoided and defended against. It is true that these executives have been rewarding themselves for years for doing nothing and they have done the same thing, stealing from the owners (the shareholders) of the corporation. This idea could be turned around so that the board are the greedy thieves. Even so that would make them even more convenient repositories for his projected greedy oral sadism.

What is so striking about this speech is Gekko's prideful public assertion that greed is good. This is in contrast to how we typically view greed: greed is bad. After all, greed, defined as acquiring more wealth than one needs is one of the seven deadly sins and is considered a "sin against God." Webster's International Dictionary (1971) similarly defines greed as inordinate or all consuming, as a reprehensible acquisitiveness for wealth and gain, and as an extreme or voracious desire for food and drink. Implicit in this definition is the notion that greed is reprehensible if it is directed toward wealth and gain, but not necessarily if it involves a food and drink, then suggests that we are much more forgiving of voracious appetites for food or drink than for money.

Madoff concealed his greed. It was hidden behind his reserved withdrawn, personality, and masked by his charitable gifts, and board seats in well-respected organizations. As Kaplan (1991) points out, even the Hunt brothers, who showed little compunction in attempting to corner the silver and then the soybean market, tried to maintain a public façade of concern for their victims to hide the sadistic pleasure they took in hurting and bankrupting them.

Gekko is different; in the speech he proudly proclaims the value of greed, ". . . greed is good, greed works, greed is right, greed clarifies, cuts through and captures the essence of the evolutionary spirit. Greed in all its forms has marked the upward surge of mankind and greed, mark my words, will save not only Teldar Paper [the company he is trying to take over], but that other malfunctioning corporation called the U.S.A."

After the speech the stockholders rise, cheer, and applaud. In the moment, they idealize and identify with Gekko, imagining that they too can become the omnipotent, powerful and wealthy Gekko, who serves as an idealized authority figure gives them permission to allow their greedy fantasies to emerge into consciousness in full force. An exciting group mania takes hold but, like a transference cure, the mania cannot be sustained without the continued incorporation of the idealized object. Eventually it will dissipate as the limitations of reality set in, internal sanctions re-emerge, and the recognition of harm done to others becomes unavoidable. None of us is immune from the temptation to actualize master of the universe fantasies of unlimited power and wealth. But we also realize that the unfettered actualization of such fantasies undermines, rather than supports, the evolutionary process and brings untold harm.

We are then left with the dilemma of finding a useful place for greed; greed that is adaptive, and normal, greed that can be transformed into healthy strivings to benefit both individuals and society. What are the defining characteristics of good greed, and are we even justified in calling it greed? Greed is typically understood as all-consuming, voracious, reprehensible, and insatiable. Good greed has none of these qualities. Perhaps we should restrict our definition of greed to bad greed and define good greed as healthy self-assertion. Such a definition would capture important essential elements of good greed, but in my view would serve a defensive function, sanitizing our conscious and unconscious fantasies and moving us away from our biological and evolutionary heritage. This makes it all the more important to distinguish good greed from bad greed and integrate good greed in our understanding of personality functioning.

Good greed, unlike bad greed, emerges out of optimal experiences of frustration and gratification and is balanced by love and recognition of the wholeness, separateness, and subjectivity of the other. Envy is always present stimulating greed, but it is not fused with sadistic fantasies and the need to spoil and take revenge. Instead, envy serves as a catalyst for strivings for realistic goals. And perhaps most importantly, in good greed, strivings for power and control are not employed in the service of sustaining defensive omnipotent fantasies transformed into beliefs about self. Rather they are integrated into adaptive strivings tempered by realistic limitations, internal evolved moral constraints, and by an awareness of their impact on self and other.

REFERENCES

ABRAHAM, K. (1924). *The Influence of Oral Eroticism on Character Formation. In On Character and Libido Frustration.* New York: Norton 1966.

BALINT, M. (1952). On Love and Hate. *International Joural of Psychoanalysis* 33:355–362.

HORNEY, K. (1937). *The Neurotic Personality of Our Time.* New York: Norton.

——— (1950). Neurosis and Human Growth. New York: Norton.

JOSEPH, B. (1960). Some Characteristics of the Psychopathic Personality, *International Journal of Psychoanalysis* 41:526–531.

KAPLAN, H.A. (1991). Greed: A Psychoanalytic Perspective. *Psychoanalytic Review,* 78:505–523.

KLEIN, M. (1957). Envy and Gratitude, London: Tavistock.

STANLEY, A. (2008). Scandals to Warm To. (2008, December 21). *The New York Times*, p. WK1 of the New York edition.

SUN-TZU (1988, T. Cleary translation). *The Art of War.* Boston, MA: Shambhala Publications.

Webster's Third New International Dictionary of the English Language Unabridged. Springfield, MA: G. & C. Merriam Company, Publishers, 1971.

Ken Winarick, Ph.D.
170 West End Avenue (#27P)
New York, NY 10023–5418
Kenwinaric@aol.com

Lawrence Josephs

CHAPTER 1

THE ADAPTIVE FUNCTION OF SEXUAL GREED

The dictionary has defined greed as excessive or reprehensible acquisitiveness. In religion, greed is considered one of the seven deadly sins. In psychoanalytic thinking, greed in adulthood is considered a persisting infantile symptom (or characteristic that must be outgrown or sublimated to enable reciprocal relationships with others characterized by caring, sharing, and mutual support.

Melanie Klein linked greed to an inborn oral insatiability in which no amount of gratification is ever quite enough. From a sociological and political point of view, greed is seen as a root cause of social injustice. An insatiable desire for money, status, and power has been thought to generate a world of "haves" and "have-nots" who have been cold-heartedly and unfairly denied their rightful due by the former.

There is no doubt that greed gets a bad rap in most traditional and contemporary discourses. The only positive reference to greed that I can recall is from Oliver Stone's movie *Wall Street* (1987) in which the protagonist Gordon Gecko proclaims that "greed is good" to a cheering crowd. In saying that greed is good Gecko is verbalizing a fallacy, the same fallacy made by the social Darwinists in the nineteenth century who misused the idea of survival of the fittest to justify social inequities. Ruthless acquisitiveness may be an inherent aspect of human nature that has evolved through natural selection. By the same token, social cooperation and the sharing of resources may also be an inherent aspect of human nature that has evolved through natural selection. So that an innate part of human nature is the conflict between greedy acquisitiveness and the spontaneous impulse to share our resources based upon empathic identification with the needs of others.

We see spontaneous sharing at a young age when two-year olds spontaneously share their food in trying to feed their parents or to feed animals at a petting zoo. Yet we also see greedy covetousness when children try to grab toys away from other children and try to keep them all to themselves. Researchers have begun to look at emotions from an evolutionary point of view and to assume that all emotions evolve to serve adaptive functions. (Oatley et al., 2006) From this point of view, emotions are species characteristic response patterns that are designed to solve particular families of adaptive problems encountered in what Bowlby (1972) called the environment of evolutionary adaptedness. To the extent that human greed is a universal aspect of human nature, it would seem to be designed to confront some long-standing evolutionary problem to which humans were required to adapt over the course of evolution. Similarly, the emotions that support cooperative sharing of resources are also designed to confront some long-standing evolutionary problem.

Before delving into the specific adaptive function of greed in humans and of sexual greed in particular we must understand how contemporary evolutionary biologists have developed a different but complementary way of understanding the concept of adaptation from the one that psychoanalysts usually use. Hartmann (1958) articulated an adaptive viewpoint in order to link psychoanalysis and biology. Hartmann wrote, "We call a man well-adapted if his productivity, his ability to enjoy life, and his mental equilibrium are undisturbed" (Ash & Gallup,.2008).

Evolutionary psychologists have critiqued this view of adaptation because it assumes that "psychological mechanisms would evolve merely to achieve mental relief, regardless of the utility of the actions they motivated (Barash & Lipton, 2001).

> Contrary to what many people have been taught, evolution has nothing to do with the survival of the fittest. It is not a question of whether you live or die. The key to evolution is reproduction. Whereas all organisms eventually die, not all organisms reproduce. Organisms do not compete among themselves for scarce resources or survival. Rather, they compete for genetic representation in subsequent generations. . . . As a consequence, what is or is not adaptive has to be measured in terms of its impact on reproduction. An adaptive trait is one that confers a reproductive advantage. (Bowlby, 1972).

Psychoanalysts tend to look at adaptation in more proximate terms such as how a psychological trait contributes to maintaining homeostatic balance or relational connections in the here-and-now. They (We) look at human sexuality and appreciate the multiple functions that it serves such as gratifying the desire for sexual pleasure, establishing a relational connection, boosting self-esteem, or, on occasion making a baby. In contrast, evolutionary psychologists look at adaptation in distal terms—how a trait ultimately confers a reproductive advantage over the course of evolution, perhaps at the expense of mental well-being, relational security, or even individual survival. For example, a peacock's bright feathers are a sexually selected trait that confers a reproductive advantage but because it makes it easier to spot by predators, may constitute a disadvantage in terms of individual survival.

Adaptation for an evolutionary biologist means discovering how a trait evolved as a strategy for reproductive advantage. For example, oral greediness might evolve not simply to insure individual survival but to increase reproductive success, Better fed individuals may seem like more desirable sexual partners, may be more fertile, may have sufficient food to sire a greater number of offspring, might be able to raise better fed children and grandchildren, may have longer lives thus being able to better support children and grandchildren and might be able to build stronger coalitions because of their ability to distribute excess resources to hungry others. Therefore oral greediness could translate not only into better prospects for individual survival but also into better prospects for reproductive success. Oral greed evolves as an adaptation for reproductive advantage if orally greedy individuals sire more and healthier offspring than less greedy individuals.

Yet oral greed would diminish over the course of evolution if sharing food with non-kin who reciprocate the favor leads to better reproductive outcome in the long-term. Then it may become adaptive to punish orally greedy individuals who refuse to share their food or who steal other people's food. If empathy with the hunger of others isn't enough to inspire equitable distribution of food, the fear of being punished for being orally greedy might inspire people to share resources despite their inclinations to be withholding.

For evolutionary biologists adaptation is not necessarily synonymous with what is morally good, with what leads to homeostatic balance, with what leads to social adjustment, or even with what leads to individual survival. For evolutionary biologists, adaptation is simply whatever reproductive strategy has led to reproductive success in the environment even if that reproductive strategy makes the individual absolutely miserable, hurts a lot of other people, and causes an early death.

Is sexual greed as an adaptation for reproductive advantage? Can we be greedy when it comes to sex? Can our sexuality be excessive and reprehensibly acquisitive? Is sexual possessiveness of our partners a form of greediness and is sexually sharing our partners a form of generosity? Is the desire for an endless variety of sexual partners a form of greed whereas restriction us to monogamous arrangements a form of equitable distribution of sexual resources? Are there sexual "haves," and sexual "have knots"? Do the sexually greedy rationalize and hide their sexual greediness to avoid punishment by those who believe that sexual resources should be equitably and fairly distributed? Sexual greed becomes a highly charged issue once we consider the possibility that sex may be considered a limited resource? Some sexual partners are considered more desirable than others making the most sexually desirable partners a scarce resource. As a consequence, some will have greater access to more desirable partners than others.

Those who are good at monopolizing sexual resources can be greedy, leaving the rest feeling unfairly sexually deprived. What seems to be the patently unfair but stark reality of the sexual marketplace is that individuals perceived as young, beautiful, affluent, smart, funny, confident, outgoing, and caring generally possess higher mate value than individuals perceived as old, ugly, poor, dumb, insecure, introverted, and uncaring (Buss, 2003). Individuals with the highest mate value can monopolize sexual resources greedily while those with the lowest mate value may be left in the sexual poorhouse. The ways in which these issues play out in our patients' presenting problems are almost clichés. The typical sexual "have-nots" may be single heterosexual women whose biological clocks are running out and who complain about the dearth of single men suitable for a long-term committed relationship or divorced middle- aged women who complain that men their own age only want significantly younger women. Sexually frustrated young adult heterosexual males complain that casual sex appears to be a scarce resource while middle-aged men without significant financial resources complain that women reject them because they don't make enough money. Similarly, middle-aged gay men complain that they have neither the looks nor the money to attract the younger gay men to whom they are sexually attracted.

We may also work with the sexual" haves" who have to cope with the spoiling envy and moralistic aggression of those who object to their sexually privileged position. There are the young, handsome, and successful gay and straight men who readily gratify their desires for casual sex with a wide variety of partners, the overwhelming majority of whom will be rejected as not good enough for a long-term relationship. There are young beautiful women who monopolize heterosexual male attention while less attractive women fail to inspire the reflexive "attentional adhesion" of the average heterosexual male to whom they have become invisible. There are unfaithful married individuals with children who try to enjoy the emotional security of monogamous family life while surreptitiously enjoying the sexual freedoms of a single individual. Their only problem is dealing with the rage of their spouses when caught cheating and/or the fury of their frustrated lovers whom they disappoint by not leaving their spouses.

We are all sexually greedy, at least in fantasy, but it would seem that only those perceived as high in mate value are readily afforded the opportunity to indulge their sexual greediness in real life and, if lucky, evade the penalties. As a consequence, those perceived as possessing lower mate value are often left feeling unfairly sexually deprived as well as shamefully inferior. Those with lower apparent mate value may be left with the sour grapes of sore losers so respond enviously and moralistically to the seemingly lucky few who can gratify their sexual greed to the hilt, seemingly without suffering any adverse consequences.

To understand how sexual greed can be adaptive from an evolutionary point of view, we have to understand the concept of reproductive strategies in evolutionary biology. Quantity-over-quality reproductive strategies are strategies in which individuals try to sire large number of offspring with minimal parental investment. The assumption is that only the hardiest offspring will survive and there may be high infant mortality. More effort is put into mating, acquiring the good genes of hardy individuals, than into parenting. Quality over quantity reproductive strategies are strategies in which individuals limit the number of offspring and increase the parental investment in order to achieve a higher rate of infant survival. Less effort is put into mating and more effort is put into parenting.

The evolution of internal gestation and lactation among mammals meant that mammalian females evolved towards a quality-over-quantity strategy (Hrdy, 1999). Among primates this tendency increased as primate females tend to only have one birth at a time unlike dogs or cats which routinely have multiple births and let the runt of the litter perish. Primates, like chimpanzees and presumably humans, probably only had a single offspring once every three years in the environment of evolutionary adaptedness since lactation suppresses ovulation so that a new offspring is not conceived until its older sibling has been weaned.

In contrast, the majority of male mammals continued to pursue a quantity over quality strategy, putting almost all energy into competing with other males for access to multiple partners and almost no effort into paternal care. Yet around five percent of mammals in contrast to eighty percent of birds have evolved in a more monogamous direction in order to facilitate biparental care (Barash & Lipton, 2001). Monogamy is a quality-over-quantity reproductive strategy. Human males have thus moderated the strategy of the typical mammalian male in order to invest highly in a smaller number of offspring Females have had to alter their reproductive strategies as males evolved towards monogamous investments. When all males are promiscuous and there is no possibility of paternal care, the challenge for females is to be inseminated by "good genes." There are the genes of the hardiest and healthiest males, often those best able to win competitive contests, be they contests of physical strength, skill, or beauty. The point is to sire as many genetically healthy and hardy offspring as possible and to achieve genetic diversification of offspring by having offspring sired by different fathers of high genetic quality. As men become monogamously inclined, females must compete among one another for the men who will be the most devoted fathers and the best providers, regardless of whether they possess other desirable genetically heritable qualities. Monogamy requires that women sacrifice genetic diversification of offspring by siring all offspring with just one man of perhaps only average genetic quality. Monogamously oriented men seem most willing to commit to the healthiest most fertile looking women they can attract requiring some women to compete in beauty contests for male attention.

Though we sometimes think of these gender differences as arbitrary social constructions, evolutionary psychologists have begun to think of culture as a vehicle of sexual selection. For example, ochre which is used for red cosmetic adornment is one of the oldest cultural artifacts in the archaeological record suggesting that one aspect of culture, physical adornment, may have been driven by a competition for sexual selection. The "sham menstruation" hypothesis speculates that red cosmetic adornment symbolically simulates menstrual blood, and menstruation was a reliable cue to imminent fertility in an environment of evolutionary adaptedness because menstruation was a relatively rare event when most fertile women are either pregnant or lactating. (Power, 1999) Thus fashion conscious early humans may have been more successful in reproducing than those who were not able to adorn themselves to enhance their mate value. It may not be so much that culture constructs our sexuality but rather that we construct culture in order to advance our reproductive self-interests. We cultivate and advertise our artistic, musical, or literary talents because we appreciate intuitively that displaying our capacity to construct meaningful cultural artifacts during romantic courtship is an inherently sexy trait. (Miller, 2000) We may construct sexual moralities as a means of thwarting the successful implementation of reproductive strategies that seem to threaten our own.

Sex differences in mating strategies appear to generate sex differences in sexual greed. Greedy heterosexual men oriented towards a quantity over quality reproductive strategy appear to want infinite sexual variety with a never-ending stream of sexually indulgent women. Pornography seems to cater to that insatiable male fantasy. Greedy heterosexual men oriented towards a quality over quantity reproductive strategy hope to win the ultimate trophy woman, a perfect 10, as a soul mate with whom they will live happily ever after and have high paternal investment in a limited number of children. Greedy heterosexual men who want the best of both worlds hope to form large harems thereby entirely shutting out subordinate men from the mating market. Harems enable men to possess and monopolize sexually a large number of desirable women who will not be shared with other men. Such men will sire many children, though there may be high paternal investment in just a few favorites. Wealthy men in modern monogamous societies who divorce middle-aged wives in order to sire more offspring with younger women try to achieve in the modern world what only despots could achieve in the ancient world.

Sexually greedy heterosexual women want to win as monogamous partners greedy men who successfully monopolize economic resources. The greater resources a man has to invest in his children, the better the rate of survival and future reproductive prospects of a woman's children, and the more children she can afford to bear and raise in an advantaged environment. When men with economic resources are a scarce commodity as in the inner city, sexually greedy women may start having children at a young age, bearing children with different fathers by getting impregnated by the sexiest men that they can attract despite middle-class disapproval. Though not often acknowledged, modern women may still be unconsciously shopping around to be inseminated with superior genes. Women, single as well as married, may be oriented towards casual sex with handsome studs so as to sire the offspring of healthy and hardy men, even if such men do not offer the possibilities of much paternal investment. It has been estimated that from 10– to 15% of men may be unknowingly raising children who are not their own. (Cerda-Flores et al, 1999) Women of independent means or who have childcare help from maternal kin may be less reliant on men for resources. Therefore they are freer to pursue a strategy of acquiring the best genes and can obtain the reproductive benefits of genetic diversification by bearing the offspring of different men with good genes. Since younger men generally have higher quality sperm, less likely to result in birth defects than that of older men, older women with declining fertility might be motivated to mate with desirable younger men who are at the height of their fertility.

It seems likely that there is a universal belief that our offspring will resemble our sexual partners in terms of both physical and mental characteristics. Strength of sexual attraction is to some extent an unconscious barometer of how much we would implicitly like to produce offspring who possess the traits to which we are sexually attracted With the advent of modern reproductive technology people try to be as choosey as they can about the physical and mental characteristics of the egg and sperm donors with whom they attempt to reproduce.

Sexual greed is a high- risk, high- gain reproductive strategy since indulging our sexual greed exposes us to the spoiling envy and moralistic aggression of those who feel that we are taking more than our fair share at their expense. Poaching other people's sexual partners, cheating on our own sexual partners, trying to monopolize more than one sexual partner, wanting casual sex with an endless variety of desirable sexual partners without ever making a commitment to any of them, men having offspring with different women whom they do not parent or support, and women having offspring with a variety of sexy men who offer little paternal support may all be forms of sexual greed that arouse the spoiling envy and moralistic aggression of others whose own sexual greed has been denied. (How about the cost to society both economically and socially?) The children of the sexually greedy may resent not being the recipients of exclusive bi-parental care and having to share limited parental resources not only with full siblings but with half siblings, step-siblings, step-parents, and the parents' other lovers. Most cultures reinforce moral condemnation of sexually greedy behavior, though there are subcultures in which certain forms of sexual greed are considered normal especially for high status men.

Limiting our sexual greed is a low risk low gain reproductive strategy. By limiting our love lives to a single partner of mate value roughly equivalent to our own and to whom we remain loyal and devoted, we evade the potentially high costs of being exposed to the spoiling envy and moralistic aggression of others. The cost is lost mating opportunities. We limit our sexual satisfactions as well as our ultimate reproductive success in terms of the quantity, genetic quality, and genetic diversification of our offspring. Yet we may try to compensate for some of those costs through high parental investment from both parents in which heroically self-sacrificing attempts are made to enable a few genetically similar offspring to live up to their fullest potential regardless of their inherent limitations.

These are extremely touchy issues to raise without provoking self-righteous moral indignation. It severely wounds our narcissism to think of ourselves as sexually greedy individuals who may possess low inherent mate value and are, therefore full of spoiling envy and moralistic rage, towards individuals who are more sexually desirable, sexually fulfilled, and reproductively successful. Yet I think that when we fail to raise such issues we are leaving an aspect of our repudiated narcissistic aspirations unanalyzed and an unconscious source of exquisite shame and guilt. A retired Jewish female patient of mine was conflicted about moving to a retirement community in Florida. She had never married or had children and was mortified by the thought of sitting around the pool while everybody bragged about the successes of their children and grandchildren. Yet she hated herself for vindictively wanting to withhold the mirroring validation to which these reproductively successful senior citizens felt narcissistically entitled. She felt that as because she had lost the mating game, she had become an invisible woman. On rare occasion when people did see her as a real person she felt shamed because she felt that people looked at her more with pity than with empathy or interest. Perceiving me as a smugly self-satisfied reproductive winner made it difficult to analyze this issue without seeming patronizing. Despite the difficulty, I believe that the analytic process is facilitated when patients can discuss their sexual greed, their spoiling envy of those who gratify their sexual greed, their sexually competitive preoccupation with their relative mate value, and their relative reproductive successes and failures without feeling shamed in the process for being too narcissistic.

In conclusion, let me say that I don't know whether or not these evolutionary speculations are indeed true but psychoanalysts should be aware that there is a growing body of research that supports such hypotheses. I believe that these evolutionary speculations attune us to a dimension of conscious and unconscious sexual fantasy life whose analysis is often neglected because it's too touchy an issue.

REFERENCES

ASH, J. & GALLUP, G. (2008). Brain size, intelligence, and Paleolithic variation. In *Mating Intelligence: Sex, Relationships, and the Mind's Reproductive System*, ed by Geher, G. & Miller, G. New York: Erlbaum. pp. 313–336.

BARASH, D.P. & LIPTON, J.E. (2001). *The Myth of Monogamy: Fidelity and Infidelity in Animals and People.* New York: Freeman.

BOWLBY, J. (1972). *Attachment: Attachment and Loss, Vol. 1.* Middlesex, UK: Penguin Books.

BUSS, D.M. (2003). *The evolution of desire. Revised Edition.* New York: Basic Books.

CERDA-FLORES, R. M., BARTON, S. A., MARTY-GONZALEZ, L. F., RIVAS, F., & CHAKRABORTY, R. (1999). Estimation of nonpaternity in the Mexican population of Nuevo Leon: A validation study of blood group markers. *American Journal of Physical Anthropology,* 109:281–293.

HARTMANN, H. (1958). *Ego Psychology and the Problem of Adaptation.* New York: International Universities Press.

HRDY, S.B. (1999). *Mother Nature: Maternal Instincts and How They Shape the Human Species.* New York: Ballantine Books.

MILLER, G. (2000). *The Mating Mind.* New York: Anchor Books.

OATLEY, K., KELTNER, D., & JENKINS, J.M. (2006). *Understanding Emotions: Second Edition.* Oxford, UK: Blackwell Publishing.

POWER, C. (1999). Beauty magic: The origins of art. In *The Evolution of Culture.* R. Dunbar, C. Knight, & C. Power, Eds. New Brunswick, NJ: Rutgers University Press.

Lawrence Josephs
401 East 65th Street, #2F
New York, NY 10065
josephs@adelphi.edu

Janice S. Lieberman

CHAPTER 2

Some Reflections on Greed and Envy in the "Recent" Age of Affluence

One young, well-dressed businessman to another: "There are only two kinds of people who live in New York City: the ones who get obscenely huge salaries and those who don't make enough to live even vaguely decently." He expands: "The ones who get millions of dollars in bonuses, and the others who have to struggle by on $200,000."

This exchange, noted in *The New York Times,* Metropolitan Diary (February 19, 2007) was a social reality of the past several years.

When back in 1925 F. Scott Fitzgerald wrote in *The Great Gatsby* that: "the very rich are different from you and me," he was referring to a hidden world of a privileged few that most people did not see or even read about in their daily lives. In the past ten years the socioeconomic pie has been reconfigured. Until last fall the rich were getting richer, and there were many of them, and many of them known to you and me (Frank 2007; Herbert 2007; Johnston 2007; Sorkin 2007). The media we read, e.g., *The New York Times, The Wall Street Journal,* are still replete with stories about 45 million dollar apartments, 50-million-dollar paintings, those who use their private jets to travel to their multiple homes. In our major cities live large numbers of men and women in their 20s and 30s who have earned millions in financial arenas and in the better law firms; some are already retired. They inhabit the increasing number of high-end expensive coops and condos being built, eat in four and five star restaurants, and their indifference to any thrift or questioning of bills has driven the price of everything upward in the neighborhoods in which they live. The term "affluenza" has become part of our parlance.

There is a clear demarcation between these "haves" and the "have-nots" of their own age. At this moment of time, among the "have-nots" are the higher educated university professors, scholars, scientists, doctors, psychiatrists, psychoanalysts, social workers: *ourselves and the bulk of those who we see in clinical practice.* Those among us who have in treatment a number of the "haves" privately complain to one other that their wealthier patients often present greater fee collection issues than those who do not have so much money. Some, on account of their wealth, feel entitled to withhold fees, and then make their *analysts* out to be the greedy ones, anxious to collect.

To Have and Have Not (taken from Hemingway's novel) was the title of a Panel at the Meetings of the American Psychoanalytic Association in 2000 chaired by Irene Cairo-Chiarandini 2001. There is also Kaplan's (1991) comprehensive paper on greed, which has informed this paper. Wurmser and Jurass (2008) have edited a book about jealousy and envy. But very little has been written about *greedy and envious patients*. There have been some writings on the clinical issues that arise when working with *wealthy patients* (Rothstein 1986; Warner 1991; Dimen 1994; Josephs 2004; Kirsner 2006). It has been my experience that greedy and envious patients may need many years of psychotherapy before they can be analyzed. Their greed and envy are syntonic, and the source of the difficulties they have in life are externalized for a long period of time. Their parents, spouses, even fate, are to blame for whatever misfortunes have brought them into treatment. The old fashioned term "oral-dependent character" seems to apply to them. Superego functioning may seem diminished, but I believe that we are working with "a new and different superego."

Let me give you a brief vignette describing how times and my own view of the world have changed. About ten years ago, a 40-year-old investment banker came into treatment with me. He lived in a Westchester suburb and commuted to the city for work. He discovered that his wife was having an affair. And she had asked him for a divorce. He was especially upset about having to sell his home, and about dividing of his wealth. He cried because he was afraid that his daughter would no longer be popular at school without the separate playhouse she had on their current property. He believed strongly that with less money he could not possibly attract the kind of woman he desired—a physical "ten." At that time I had difficulty imagining or relating to his world. It was difficult to feel empathic with this man in order to really help him. Ten years later, the media, and what I have personally witnessed in my private life and have heard from my patients, have made it so that I can imagine it.

Today's psychoanalysts can no longer consider themselves to be upper echelon earners, if we ever were. The realities of managed care, medication as a solution to dysphoria, a world in which people have little time for personal introspection, are some of the factors that have reduced the number of hours that psychoanalysts can book. Today psychoanalysts have reason to worry about having enough patients, although we may use a certain amount of denial in order to not ruin our days (see Dimen 1994; Josephs 2004). Furthermore, our ability to accrue wealth is limited by the number of hours we work. But many of our patients have real opportunities to amass wealth. Some have no wish to amass wealth. And some, for neurotic reasons, do not pursue wealth, even when they wish to. Warner (1991) has addressed this topic directly. There is potential for serious countertransference acting out. He notes that: "most analysts have middle-class origins. They may share in the frequently found middle-class covert hatred or envy of the rich. . . . To cover it up the analyst can either show a reaction formation and be excessively ingratiating or act out this hostility by putting down the rich patient" (p. 590).

Josephs (2004) has observed that: "It is increasingly assumed that being a psychoanalyst in the United States can no longer consistently provide for the attainment of the current normative American standard of middle class affluence" (p.391). Josephs has seen a number of young patients who do not know what to do with themselves, who are irresponsible and who rely on their parents to support the treatment. They are envious of his money. Their parents regularly inquire why the patient needs to go more than once a week. Others have parents who will not give them any money. "These patients are barely on speaking terms with their parents" (p. 400).

Most of us who conduct psychoanalysis rely on inner values and are sustained more by the quality of our relationships and experiences than we are by material things To what extent should our personal values be expressed to patients with different value systems? In a world in which those who "go for the money" are more valued than we ourselves, do we do our patients a disservice if we attempt overtly, or more likely, covertly to shape them according to the way we are? To those of us who have supported ourselves since we were in our twenties, adults who feel entitled to parental financial assistance and refuse to work, seem disturbed, and are disturbing to us. Today, women who refuse to work, and insist that their husbands support them, also seem to be disturbed. But are they not just coming with another set of cultural values? I believe that these are important issues to ponder.

Let us go back thirty years. The 1980's was a great time for Wall Street. In Oliver Stone's film by that name, the main character, Gordon

Gekko, declared that "Greed is Good" (*Wall Street* 1987) Those born between 1960 and 1980, who are roughly 30 to 50 today, grew up with a different value system. It was a time of prosperity in which there was also much self-examination. Whatever was considered sacred was being challenged: the Viet Nam war, the institution of marriage, and, in particular, gender roles. When I began my practice in the mid-seventies, anti-materialism, the "greening of America," autonomy and self-sufficiency, were valued. It was a time of feminist uprising: mothers went back to school, back to work, and some divorced. For a long time there was little or no back-up mothering. Unlike today when we have in place an army of professional care-givers, the parenting many children received was uneven, at best. Latchkey children were met at the end of the day by mothers too tired to give them needed attention. Mothers and fathers felt guilty that their children had two parents working; some were guilty that their children had to witness divorce and live in two different places. Misusing psychological and psychoanalytic advice and expertise, they often tolerated the excessive demands of their children, many of whom we are seeing today as adults in analysis and therapy. I see these childrearing facts of our recent history as sources of the greed and envy we see in our consulting rooms today.

Let me fast-forward to the first decade of the twenty-first century. The kind of separation-individuation most of us worked at in our youth is no longer the norm. Nowadays families are more often than not enmeshed. Children, adolescents and grown children dominate their parents who are fearful that their children will hate them or, especially, that they will abandon them. Whereas in the 1970s "terrorist" adolescents or twenty-somethings were involved in political causes, in this decade "terrorist" adolescents and twenty-somethings demand money and material things from their parents.

We have in our practices young adults who were both emotionally deprived and overindulged. I have coined the term "masked deprivation" to describe what I have witnessed: material things are provided but not the kind of psychological attunement needed for children to develop optimally. Many young adults today do not have the ego strength and frustration tolerance to seek work that will support them. They observe their friends' parents supporting their friends, buying them apartments, finding them jobs and partners. They do not leave home even when they have physically left home, and they are tied to their parents all day long by cell-phones, Blackberries or iPhones.

I have seen in my practice, as well as in my private life, the seduction and courting of young married couples, who are taken by the parents of one member of the couple on expensive vacations, promised country houses near these parents and many other luxuries in an effort to keep the family together and in some cases to see that the *other* family does not get to see the couple or their future children as much.

All the more problematic for psychoanalytic treatment, the parents often pay for, and thus compromise or try to control, the treatment. In his paper on the children of wealthy parents Warner (1991) wrote that "Their sense of reality can become distorted because if they get in trouble they know they will always be "bailed out" and never have to face the consequences of their actions as others do" (p. 579). They externalize, and get their doctors to tell them what they want to hear. "Another significant transference problem is the attempted seduction of the analyst through the affluent patient's money, charm or power" (p. 590). As we know, Freud himself was not immune to this as he sought funds to support his psychoanalytic endeavors. As Kirsner, D.(2007) noted, in his paper entitled "Do as I say, not as I do: Ralph Greenson, Anna Freud, and superrich patients," Greenson, who wrote a Bible of proper technique , not only stretched the boundaries with Marilyn Monroe, but with a number of superrich patients, all of this taking place with Anna Freud"s knowledge and approval.

Those of my own patients, and these are still the bulk of my practice, whose parents were able to cut the emotional and financial umbilical cord when they graduated from college seem not to be plagued by these issues. They found jobs; their conflicts in work or love are not encumbered by this order of envy or greed. I can describe them as having fiber, *moral fiber*, mature consciences and superegos, just what that seems to be lacking in the group I am speaking about. Intersecting with this is the early onset of sexual activity. Young people today sometimes have their first sexual encounter at 12 or 13, and are encouraged to sleep with their partners in their parents' houses. They often have a strict sense of morality, swearing "fidelity" to the person they have slept with before getting to know that person. There is a lack of consequences for laziness, for aggression toward elders, for having sex at a young age.

Despite the considerable advances women have made in the world at large, some of my young women patients seem to be in particular difficulty. Over-gratification and prolonged dependency on parents has resulted in their limited acquisition of basic skills for functioning independently: cooking, furnishing a home, purchasing clothing, paying bills. We have a generation of young women who hire lactation specialists to help them nurse; specialists to plan weddings, wrap gifts, set tables, choose colors for rooms; personal shoppers to choose a wardrobe and create their "style"; and personal assistants to do it all. Spas have multiplied, as this generation demands constant soothing and massage of every part of their bodies as a way of coping with poor anxiety tolerance, the end result of early over-gratification and neglect. Coupled with this is the expectation that they have successful careers and gorgeous homes, that they look perfect and have perfect bodies, requiring hours at the gym and rigorous dieting, further reducing their energy.

In my book *Body Talk: Looking and Being Looked at in Psychotherapy* (2000), in a way a precursor to this paper, I cited Brumberg (1997), who found that contemporary adolescent girls' diaries were filled with the self-critical phrase "I'm so ugly." She compared these with the writings of nineteenth century girls, who valued "good works". Brumberg noted that: "Before World War I, girls rarely mentioned their bodies in terms of strategies for self-improvement or struggles for personal identity. Becoming a better person meant paying *less* attention to the self, giving more assistance to others" (p. xxi). In the recent Presidential election, Obama was photographed in his daily "workout," breaking a sweat, as a way of appealing to this imperative. He was described as "religiously" devoted to his exercise. Sarah Palin proudly announced that she hid her recent pregnancy until the seventh month because she had "tight abs."

Some of the young men I have seen in my practice have suffered from having had parents who were often absent when they needed them, but who now expect them, as young adults, to achieve. They are watched over like hawks, and at the first sign of faltering, their parents take over, writing applications to colleges for them, making phone calls and pulling strings to get them jobs. These efforts are not private, but public, and the young men exchange the shame of potential failure for the shame of letting their parents take over their lives for them; all the while, their parents are telling their friends and relatives of their efforts on behalf of their sons. One male patient, 45 years old, spent hours on the phone with his mother, who counseled every minute of his business deal hoping that his business success would take him off the dole. It is my contention that the exact opposite effect would happen.

At this juncture one can ask just what is greed? And what makes an analyst think that his patient is greedy? The assessment of greed from manifest content is problematic because it is so culture and value system specific. "Affluence" is also culture-specific. I recall a supervisor of mine in the early 70s calling a patient of mine "greedy" because she and her friends celebrated her birthday at an expensive restaurant. I had assessed this as finally "letting herself have things"! Paradoxically when I needed another control case this same supervisor referred for analysis an educated young man who arrived wearing a t-shirt that said "OUTRAGEOUS." He hoped to pay me $5 a session and to come four day per week. He was a graduate student who was about to marry a wealthy woman. Her father was paying for their honeymoon, doing the Grand Tour of Europe and staying in posh hotels, and had also purchased an apartment for them. He had no plans to work for years.

What happens in the treatment when the analyst's values, the analyst's notions of what is right or wrong, are very different from those of the patient? It creates a complication in the analysis.

A wealthy woman patient, Susan, appears every week with a different handbag, each in the $2,000 to $10,000 category. Her suits, coats and furs, shoes and jewelry, all are expensive and different each week. She does not mention her purchases, when or how she made them, alone or with an advisor. I ask myself whether I am just envious to think of her as greedy. She was born into wealth. Is she not entitled to spend it? I sometimes question myself. I have a small country house. Am I greedy, having two places in which to live when there is so much poverty in the world? I think of a most hard-working therapist-patient, Bridget who wears the same pocketbook—which must have cost her $20—four days a week. Business people in New York (at least until this past October) went out for expensive dinners at which they ordered $1,000 bottles of wine. At my institute, $10 bottles of wine are served, and we are always short of money. A male patient Tom spends much time fitting his custom-made suits, shirts and shoes, sports equipment, computer toys, and regards his clothing and paraphernalia to be essential to attract the kind of women he likes to date, and for him to fit into the places he goes to. Am I envious, or is he just greedy? The technical problem with each of these patients is how to work with this issue when the patient comes from a subculture that considers this aspect of how they are living to be "just fine." And "out there" in the media, the poorly paid reporters who write for the newspapers and magazines seem to think it is "just fine" too.

Even when the patient does not consider this to be "just fine," it is difficult to work with sensitivity, and without seeming judgmental. One patient, Helen, came to treatment because of her overspending many thousands of dollars every month on clothing she did not need but was desperate for. She was particularly susceptible to the selling techniques of a luxury department store personal shopper. No amount of analysis (e.g., asking her about her thoughts, fantasies and moods just prior to a shopping spree) could enable her to check her desire. Her husband (who I suspect was having an affair) was also unable to stop her. I surmised that he tolerated it due to his own guilt, but perhaps he was as greedy as she was, and she functioned as his greedy agent.

Another patient, Eleanor, immersed in the world of "affluenza, was quite thrifty, compared with Helen, but collected large numbers of boyfriends, and binged on cookies and cake. Eating large amounts of sweets did make her feel guilty, but the other behaviors did not. Her closets were so filled with the clothes she had purchased at bargain prices that she had to rent storage space to contain some of them. The contents of her superego were very different from my own. Greed as a sin has to do with gluttony. Nevertheless, in today's world, though overeating is still a sin, purchasing four houses is a subject for admiration. "You cannot be too rich or too thin!"

I will now turn to the related topic of envy. Josephs (2004) writes: "it is vastly underreported in the clinical literature how much session time college-educated professional patients, especially in New York City, spend ventilating their financial insecurities." I agree. Every day in my practice I hear patients express envy of their wealthy parents (with Oedipal overtones), successful siblings, friends, colleagues and neighbors. A number of patients are chronically envious of me in the transference. They envy my fee, my professional standing, where my office is located, etc. The transference is difficult to analyze since there is considerable concrete reality to their complaints. Although I am aware that envy is envy despite reality, when there is a genuine difference between my reality and the patient's, it makes it difficult to get the patient to observe the transferential aspect.

It is my observation that the envy is ego-syntonic, as is the acting it out via mean, aggressive behavior toward the person who is envied. Klein (1957) noted the confusion between envy and jealousy. Envy is the earlier and more primitive affect. She defined envy as: "the angry feeling that another person possesses and enjoys something desirable – the envious impulse being to take it away or to spoil it. Moreover, envy implies the subject's relation to one person only and goes back to the earliest exclusive relationship with the mother" (Cairo-Chiarandini, 2001). Klein conceived of primary envy of the breast that is constitutive and that does not have to do with frustration (Roth and Lemma 2008). As part of the death instinct there is envy of the breast's "intolerable goodness." Envy arises at the moment when "good" is "not-me." Klein viewed greed as mainly bound up with introjection, and envy as mainly bound up with projection. Kaplan's (1991) reading of Klein is that "in greed, as contrasted with envy, there is much less recognition of the object and the focus is on possession and supplies. On an unconscious oral level, greed aims to suck out and devour the breast, essentially robbing it of its possessions. While envy has this aim, it additionally seeks to put bad parts of the self into the mother/breast. In this sense greed relates more to introjection and devouring mechanisms while envy is closely associated with spoiling aspects" (p. 512).

Greed and envy are mixed with one another. The envious feel empty. As they approach getting what they think they want they become so greedy that they destroy it. Boris (1990) has wisely noted that "the conversion of greed into appetite is an event of the first importance. Appetite . . . is susceptible to satisfaction. Greed is not. In greed . . . *any gratification only further stimulates the greed*" (p. 130).

Margery lied on her resume, cheated on her expense sheet, abused salespeople and employees. She had shop-lifted as a teenager and her mother acted as if she did not notice that Margery had a continual change of new clothes. She envied her sisters and most of her friends. Each and every one had all the things she wanted and that she was deprived of. For many years, the only way she was able to be with me in the room was to regard me as a "nothing," having nothing she wanted. I analyzed her sadism, her aggression gone amuck. She had no man in her life for many years. When a kind man from her past came on the scene, her sadism and greed re-emerged. She made outrageous demands of him, that he buy her jewelry, that he buy her a fur coat. He became hostile, then exploded with rage at her. They broke up and she was back to square one.

Paul grew up in a sexually charged household raised by random babysitters while both parents worked long hours, had separated, divorced, and reconciled. As an adult, he guiltlessly presented himself as a virtual terrorist; he reported savaging his mother, and gouging money from both parents for many years. He was chronically angry and unhappy, and a cocaine user. He became intensely angry when I confronted him with my observation that others his age worked for a living, for he maintained that he knew many who did not. When his parents gave him money or clothes, it was always too little and too late, not exactly what he wanted. He wanted a new desk and pointed to mine. He would not accept something cheesy like that. What kind of clothes would make him happy? Designer clothes only. His parents were afraid of him and appeased him. There were no consequences for his aggression and his greed. He suffered from painful envy of his classmates from his various schools over the years, certain that their lives were incredibly better than his own. He had nothing and they had everything. When his father had open heart surgery, he was envious of the attention he received.

His "psychological twin," Peter, aged 50, also came from a well-to-do family. He was always in some way supported by his father. He studied for many degrees and changed profession many times until he settled on a work identity as an artist. However he could not seem to find a job in the artistic profession he had settled on. Angry when I wondered why he had not chosen to get a regular job just to support himself he became indignant. "Where would I get doing that? I would just be wasting my life. I come from a life of privilege." He told his father: "Your main job should be finding me a job." In the transference he expected me to feed him by suggesting job possibilities he could spit out and reject. Both Paul and Peter came to treatment at ages when their non-productive years would serve as limits to what jobs they could hope to obtain even when well-analyzed. Many doors would be closed to them by then.

Carpy has noted that " patients who feel aggrieved are unable to mourn the loss of the good experiences they feel they ought to have had. Instead these patients stick to their bad experiences, as proof of their deprivation and their right to redress. Acceptance of the loss of the good experiences they have missed out on would mean having to face acute feelings of envy, both of the good object they should have had, and of the self they should have been. Thus, better to hate than to mourn. Viewed from this angle being aggrieved is both a narcissistic defense and a defense against awareness of envy" (Cairo-Chiarandini 2001, p. 1397).

CONCLUSION

Conducting psychoanalytic treatment with today's greedy and envious patients is a considerable challenge when the content of the analyst's superego is so very different from their patient's. The countertransference must be monitored at every session so that the analyst does not give into the temptation to say: "You are greedy," or "You are envious," or, "You should not treat your sister so badly just because she has become engaged to a wealthy man." These patients are provocative and the analyst must resist retaliating. The analyst must also not hang back with stony silence, detaching from the patient with disapproval. I have had some success when I ask the patient to anticipate the reality consequences of his behavior. "What do you think will happen if you do this?" I have asked: " How do you think (your sister) feels when you say that? Does that matter to you? I have remarked: "It might bother another person to come late for dinner at her sister's house. It does not seem to bother you. How come?" That is, I work with greed and envy by asking the patient to think about his actions and his thoughts. My stance is neutral and empathic.

Kohut (1971) made the distinction between traditional "guilty man" that Freudian psychoanalysis has been organized around, and "narcissistic man." The former has an internalized superego, formed as an outcome of the resolution of the Oedipus complex. Traditional psychoanalysis usually begins with a softening of the harsh, strict superego that punishes the person with unbearable feelings of guilt and depressive affect when he falls short of his ideals and values. We are not taught how to analyze faulty, deficient superegos. Greed and envy are on the short list of "the seven deadly sins," along with their companions: lust, gluttony, sloth, wrath and pride. By contrast, in this age of "narcissistic man" and the recent affluence, we observe a lack of guilt over greed and envy, little apology for hurting others and/or the analyst and a history of a lack of consequences for bad behavior. The outgrowth of the "age of narcissism" is an "age of entitlement." Since this kind of behavior (formerly regarded as "misbehavior") has become so prevalent, and government figures no longer provide us with role models for "good behavior," it is not really possible to label those feeling "entitled" as "the Exceptions." They are getting to be the norm.

REFERENCES

BORIS, H.N. (1990) "Identification with a vengeance" *Internationl Journal of Psychoanalyis* 71:127–140

BRUMBER, J. (1997) *The Body Project: An intimate history of American Girls.* New York Vintage Books.

CAIRO-CHIARANDINI, I. (2001). To have and have not: Clinical uses of envy. *Journal of the American Psychoanalytic Association* 49:1391–1404.

DIMEN. M. (1994). Money, love and hate: contradictions and paradox in psychoanalysis. *Psychoanalytic Dialogues* 4:69–100.

R.H. FRANK (2007). *Falling Behind: How Rising Inequality Harms The Middle Class.* New York: Basic Books)

HERBERT, B. (2007). "Nightmare before Christmas." *The New York Times* http://www.nytimes.com/2007/12/22/opinion/22herbert.html?hp

JOHNSTON, D.C. (2007). *The New York Times* 12/15/07, p. C3. "Report says that the rich are getting richer faster, much faster." http://www.nytimes.com/2007/12/15/business/15rich.html

JOSEPHS, L. (1994). Seduced by Affluence: How material envy strains the analytic relationship. *Contemporary Psychoanalysis.* 40:389–408.

KAPLAN, H. (1991) "Greed: a psychoanalytic perspective" *Psychoanalytic. Review* 78:505–523.

KIRSNER, D.(2007). "Do as I say, not as I do": Ralph Greenson, Anna Freud, and superrich patients. *Psychoanalytic Psychology* 24(3):475–486.

KLEIN, M. (1957). Envy and Gratitude: A Study of Unconscious Sources London: Tavistock Press.

KOHUT, H. (1971). *The Analysis of the Self: A Systematic Appraisal of the Psychoanalytic Treatment of Narcissistic Personalities* New York: International Universities Press.

LIEBERMAN, J.S. (2000) *Body Talk: Looking and Being Looked at in Psychotherapy* Northvale, NJ: Jason Aronson.

RIVIERE, J. (1932) "Jealousy as a mechanism of defense" in *The Inner World and Joan Riviere: Collected Papers 1920–1958,* A. Hughes ed., 1991. London: Karnac Books, Ltd., 1104–115.

ROTH, P. & LEMMA, A. (2008). *Envy and Gratitude Revisited* London: The International Psychoanalytic Association.

ROTHSTEIN, A. (1986). "The seduction of money: a brief note on an expression of transference love". Psychoan. Q. 55: 296–300.

SORKIN, A.R. *The New York Times* 12/6/07 C4 "A movie and protesters single out Henry Kravis:making an issue of private equity wealth"

WARNER, S.L. (1991) "Psychoanalytic understanding and treatment of the very rich" J. Amer. Acad. Of Psa.

WURMSER, L. & JURTASS, H., eds. (2008) *Jealousy and Envy: New Views About Two Powerful Feelings* New York and London: The Analytic Press.

Janice S. Lieberman, Ph.D.
55 East 87th Street
New York, NY 10128
JaniceLieberman@compuserve.com

Jeffrey Stern

CHAPTER 3

Oedipus or Icarus: Spitzer's Complaint or The Two Analyses of Mr. E

I need to say at the outset that talking psychoanalytically about Eliot Spitzer as I do in this paper is—as Freud wrote of our profession itself—impossible. This is because Eliot Spitzer has never been my patient. What this means is that in addition to lacking highly-detailed information about his current and early life, as well as his dreams, fantasies, fears and obsessions, I have no transference-countertransference relation to orient my understanding of him or to provide my interpretations with the sense of conviction that only being in the room with someone can make possible. What I have instead are published accounts that I have stitched together to create as whole a portrait of his personality as I can, despite the fact that little is said about his psychological life. He is thus to me more like a literary character than a "real person," and less a literary character richly drawn like Hamlet or Roskolnikov, so much as a character from a "made for TV movie" or pulp fiction or a comic book. But when I was asked if I would write about him, I assumed the point wasn't to get the real Eliot Spitzer right—I could hardly be expected to do that from Chicago where, you know, we have been occupied lately with the defrocking of a governor of our own, one whose clownish crimes had nothing to do with sex but everything to do with greed and money in accordance with our hallowed if prosaic Midwestern political traditions.

Of course we haven't only the ridiculous to think about these days in Chicago, there's also the sublime new President, Barack Obama. And the almost President and current Secretary of State Hillary Rodham Clinton. She was your Senator, New York, but she's another of our homies . . . Actually, if you think of it, Chicago is on a roll these days . . . Still, I can't believe Arnie Richards, the King or, if you prefer, Pope of Psychoanalysis, invited me to speak at this Symposium in New York! It's like being summoned to court, or Rome! Me, in New York! If I can make it there, I'll make it anywhere, bah bup bah bup New York, New York! . . . But, it makes sense he'd want a Chicago guy. Let's be honest. New York's a disaster these days now that Wall Street's collapsed. That's why the country elected Obama, a Chicago guy, to fix things. You need something done, you go to the City that Works. Arnie Richards wants a Symposium to succeed, he puts a Chicago guy on the program. Actually, I think he signed three of us! It was the same thing when New York ego psychology started to get stale. Who did Psychoanalysis turn to for new ideas? To another one of the Boyz in Mr. Obama's neighborhood, Heinz Kohut, that's who! Who's the Second City now New York? I think its time for you to take down your Manhattan-ocentric New Yorker maps and replace them with Chicago Transit Authority diagrams of the Loop . . . I have to say, with Barack in the White House its like the dawning of the Age of Michael Jordan all over again. Remember sticking it to Patrick Ewing and the Knicks year after year? How cool was that?

—Hey! Jeff! Snap out of it! What in the world are you talking about? People are waiting to hear about Eliot Sptizer! Not Barack Obama, not Rob Blagojevich, not Michael Jordan, and certainly not you!

—Uh Oh! It's my Reality Ego! And he sounds pissed! Well, so what? Why should I listen to him?

—You'd better listen, Big Shot, before they throw us both out of here!

—He's right. I have gotten side-tracked. But it's because this is so exciting. I'm not used to feeling so important. I'm about to lose control, and I think I like it!

—Nonetheless, I'm taking Jeffrey's psyche back again, and I'm going to explain that I let you, Split-off Grandiosity, lead him astray to make a point. And this is that becoming overstimulated and grandiose after being elected to high office, or after being handed billions of dollars of investors' money or for that matter after being invited to give a lecture and losing track of one's boundaries and one's mission is what this paper and I think what this Symposium is all about. And it doesn't just happen to the Eliot Spitzers and Bernard Madoffs of the world, it can happen to any of us when the moon is in the seventh house and Jupiter aligns with Mars.

—Anyway, what I was saying before beginning this lengthy digression was that when I agreed to talk about Eliot Spitzer, I assumed the point wasn't to get the real Eliot Spitzer right so much as to shed light upon the man he might be. The man he might be is enough like people we actually know and treat to make playing this game of imagining the personality of the former Governor of New York worthwhile.

So now having said all of this, "vee may," in the words of Dr. Spielvogel on the final page of *Portnoy's Complaint*, "perhaps to begin," (Roth 1969; Scheiber 2008).

Until his collapse last March, there appeared to be a single Eliot Spitzer: the righteous crusader for truth, justice and the American way. He was brilliant, aggressive, successful, perfect. He had a distinguished family, an Ivy League education, a southern belle wife and three lovely daughters. And then suddenly he was named in a sex scandal. His career flamed out like a meteor, and there were two Eliot Spitzers: the one we knew, and the one we didn't, who, as it turned out, had flown even under his family's radar for at least ten years.

Spitzer's rise and fall is the story of a boy overstimulated in childhood. His powerful father, who dreamed that Eliot would become The First Jewish President of The United States (Fineman 2008), drove him relentlessly in pursuit of this goal. He was a boy who feared his father, worrying that if he went into the real estate business Bernard Spitzer had built from nothing into a mighty empire, he would only screw things up. (Fishman 2007, p. 4.) Nonetheless, Eliot shared his father's dream of his becoming a great man, a dream shared as well by his English-professor mother.

The standard approach to such a story would follow Freud's line in his essay "Those Wrecked by Success." Spitzer's fall would be viewed as caused by unconscious guilt resulting from his attainment of the office of Governor, an achievement he would unconsciously regard as an Oedipal victory over his father (Freud 1916, pp. 315–331). Freud would have seen Spitzer's use of prostitutes as compounding his Oedipal crime by unconsciously representing the fulfillment of his desire to possess his forbidden mother. He would argue that Spitzer's vigorous effort to jail prostitution- ring leaders while he was Attorney General was his way of managing the guilt he felt over his own whoring. Katha Pollitt, writing in *The Nation,* compares Spitzer to Shakespeare's hypocritical Angelo in *Measure for Measure*, who is charged with cleaning up Vienna's licentiousness until he is discovered indulging in the very activities he is supposed to abolish (Pollitt 2008, p. 1). Freud would say that when Spitzer became Governor his Oedipal guilt became unbearable; to relieve it, he set about purposefully, if unconsciously, to give up the new office by getting himself busted in precisely the sort of prostitution sting he'd designed himself while Attorney General. He is, thus, his own worst enemy, "hoisted with his own petard" and brought to justice by his own super ego, the real sheriff of his own private Wall Street.

There may be another—doubtless there is more than one other—way to think about the rise and fall of Eliot Spitzer. If Mr. E were Mr. Z—and Heinz Kohut were analyzing him according to the model we have been discussing—the model of Mr. Z's classical first analysis—E would work through his oedipal wishes and fears until, as a result of making the unconscious conscious, he would let go of them. He would, as it were, "grow up," (Kohut 1979). Renouncing his whores, he would return to his wife and become the dutiful husband he had always pretended to be, working hard to make people forget that he had ever misbehaved. But after four or five years he would contact Kohut and say that he wasn't getting much pleasure out of his work. He had become an online journalist—and that although he had been faithful to his wife, he was feeling the pull of his old impulses. He feared that he would be unable to prevent himself from acting on them. Kohut would suggest that he return for more analysis and a different, and perhaps more sympathetic, picture of his life and personality would begin to emerge.

Of course this could never happen because Spitzer, we are told, has a Bush-like distrust of psychological thinking and he would have avoided analysts like the plague. But as that very Bush has taught us never to let facts deter us, we shall soldier on with our fantasy nonetheless. In a long profile in *The New Yorker*, Nick Paumgarten sees Spitzer as brilliant but shallow (Paumgarten 2007, p. 3), which shouldn't be all that surprising given that people who act out sexually tend—as Slavoj Zizac has said—to "enjoy their symptom[s]" too much to explore their deep meanings and risk having to give them up. (Zizac 2001). Paumgarten remembers Spitzer disdainfully asking him when they first met if he was going to write about his childhood (Paumgarten, p. 3). Indeed in the articles I've read, it isn't Spitzer but other family members and friends who remember his childhood. William Taylor, his roommate at Princeton, recalls the famous Spitzer family dinners at which Eliot the youngest, an older sister who is a lawyer, and a brother who is a neurosurgeon—were compelled by their tycoon father to debate the social issues of the day as if they were arguing before the Supreme Court. Taylor remembers worrying that he would make a fool of himself before Bernard Spitzer whom he describes as "terrifying." Paumgarten notes that Eliot was an outstanding athlete excelling at tennis and soccer but that his parents recall attending his games or matches only once while he was in high school. (White 2009). Taylor further remembers Spitzer's mother saying, on an occasion when he and Eliot had played tennis together, that she hoped he'd kicked her son's ass (Fishman 2007, p. 2). This doesn't sound like the sort of thing Oedipal mothers are supposed to say even in jest. Evidently she could see that Eliot's grandiosity—something she had doubtless contributed to—needed taming. Perhaps she also realized at some level that her son's arrogance may have masked a deep childhood depression*

Indeed, we might imagine that although he was privileged, and cherished, he was nonetheless an unmirrored child. This seems absurd on its face given that he was constantly in the spotlight at home, the impression one gets reading the accounts of these early years is that he was always in training to be the GREAT MAN his father needed him to become. It appears that he was never encouraged to feel that his parents simply loved him for himself rather than because he was the apotheosis of their narcissistic dreams. Chez Spitzer, Paumgarten dryly notes "was not an emotionally indulgent household" (Paumgarten p. 3).

Of course Eliot was nothing if not compliant. He got spectacular grades at Horace Man Preparatory School and was Student Body President at Princeton, where he is remembered not for leading sit-ins but for playing squash with the University President (Paumgarten, p. 4). But there was always a quality of bullying aggressiveness about Spitzer, an insistence that people not lead nor even follow but simply get out of his way. Indeed when he became New York State's Attorney General he famously characterized himself as a "steam roller" who would flatten his enemies like cartoon pancakes (Paumgarten, p. 2). He was loud, impatient, impetuous and easily angered, temperamentally more Shakespeare's Hotspur than the precise and bloodless Angelo,

*Howard Fineman writing in *Newsweek* recalls that he "identified something vaguely melancholy and rueful about the guy" (Fineman, 08).

because always teetering on the edge of loss of control. Perhaps there had long been a part of him that was frustrated and angry at the way he had been required to perform for the parents who had little interest in responding to what Winnicott would have called his early omnipotent gestures (Newman 1996).

Arnold Goldberg would see Spitzer's frustration as having given rise to a vertical split in his psyche which would have walled off his wounded infantile grandiosity from his "reality ego" making it impervious to the kind of taming or annealing that Ann Spitzer thought would improve him (Goldberg 1995, p. 14). Goldberg sees people with vertical splits as "being of two minds," the split-off sector often completely antithetical morally to that of the every day reality ego (Goldberg 1995, p. 14; Goldberg 1999, p. 30). A person under the moonlit sway of this split-off "other self" is aware that he may be living in utter disregard of the values he holds by day, but he seems, at least temporarily, not to care. These people know their acting out self is part of them—they aren't consciously Dr. Jekyll and unconsciously Mr. Hyde—but it somehow feels to them nevertheless that the being who violates their cherished values is someone else.

Split-off grandiosity is the sort of thing that gets politicians—and the rest of us for that matter—into trouble, because there is something somewhat psychotic about it. This is because it retains its primitive, infantile quality of absolute omnipotence. What this means is that when this aspect of the personality is in charge, we imagine ourselves more or less invulnerable and, hence, above the law. This is why someone as bright as Eliot Spitzer might do something as stupid as allowing himself to be trapped in a prostitution drag net. Or why, for that matter, Bill Clinton might think he could carry on an affair with a White House intern in the Oval Office and no one would notice. From the Kohutian-Goldbergian perspective they weren't trying unconsciously to get caught to assuage their punitive super egos, they were simply unable to engage their ordinary discretion when acting out. But why did they act out? The answer is that acting out wards-off depression, or quiets the overstimulation that in narcissistically vulnerable people may follow success.

Goldberg's idea is that the child's frustrated early need for maternal responsiveness leads to an inability to regulate self esteem in the face of narcissistic injuries. When derivatives of these early needs go unmet, they may be erotized and give rise to sexual acting out (Goldberg 1995, pp. 11–28)—This would explain Spitzer's reliance on prostitutes, a subject, that has generated a great deal of heated speculation in the ranks of the talking heads and pundits. Dr. Laura shocked Meredith Viera on *The Today Show* by suggesting that Spitzer's whoring was traceable to his wife's failure to make him feel like a man in the bedroom (Stanley 2008), an opinion echoed by a number of blogging working girls, while a writer for *New York Magazine* (Weiss 2008, p.1) judged that Spitzer simply had too much libido for one woman to satisfy, adding that any married man worth his salt shares the frustration of Spitzer's complaint. I've not been able to find much out about Silda Spitzer. She is proud of the fact that her name is a shortened version of Serilda, Teutonic for Warrior Goddess, and is described as gracious, and beautiful, a wife perfectly suited to smooth out her husband's rough edges (Fermino 2008). Their friends like her very much and were shocked to learn of Eliot's philandering given their view of the soundness of the marriage (Thomas et al. 2008). Silda has said that she liked out earning Eliot when she was a partner at Scadden, Arps and he was laboring in the public sector and that she was reluctant to give up her career to help him manage his (Paumgarten 2007, p. 3). After doing so she started a foundation to encourage rich kids such as her own to stop having outrageously expensive birthday parties and to give some of their, or their parents' money, to children who might actually need it. In this public spiritedness she is reminiscent of her mother-in-law who strove to instill in Eliot and his siblings the importance of giving back to society (White 2009).

We all probably remember Silda's impersonation of Hillary Clinton's impersonation of Tammy Wynette and standing by her man on the day that Eliot announced he was stepping down from his post in Albany. But was she a bad wife, as Dr. Laura suggests, or was the problem Eliot's unmanageable libido? Or was it something else? We have no reason to think Silda Spitzer wasn't a good wife. Her husband describes her as a person on whose judgment he absolutely relied and whom he trusted, but then, of course, Bill Clinton respected Hillary's intellect and judgment. This was evidently insufficient to keep him in her bed. The fact is we simply have no idea how gratifying a conjugal life the Spitzers enjoyed, or how much libido either partner was blessed or cursed with or without. What we know is that Eliot Spitzer began using prostitutes ten years before he was discovered to be Kristin's Client Number 9. At that time, the couple had three small daughters. If they were like other couples with small children, they probably had less time for lovemaking than they had before. Which might or might not have anything to do with Eliot's whoring. That there are records of his using prostitutes that date from this time doesn't obviate the possibility that he had been seeing prostitutes before the children were born or even before he and Silda ever met.

We also know that Client Nine required Kristen to cope with what Goldberg refers to as "the problem of perversion," meaning that he didn't simply want missionary sex, he wanted something he may have been ashamed to ask for at home. Something the capable Kristen has said she in fact didn't think a problem at all. I don't know whether Spitzer and Silda engaged in whatever it was he did with Kristen—who wasn't one to kiss and tell. It seems that a second sex worker Spitzer allegedly knew, one as it turns out who also called herself Kristen (actually Kristin) did, charging that the Governor liked it rough, (Pearson and Standora, 2009) a claim borne out by a third prostitute who told reporters that Spitzer liked role-playing games and choked her during sex (Rush and Molloy 2009). But even if Eliot and Silda did engage in the whatever-it-was, he surely couldn't have demanded that she do it whenever he may have needed it to salve his wounded narcissism after a defeat or quiet his exultation after a victory. But even if she was willing to do the "whatever" whenever, she still might have failed to provide what he needed, because Silda, the Warrior Goddess, was his partner, a companion for the parts of his personality capable of engaging another with wants and needs, likes and dislikes of her own. Given her pleasure in her name, we might be tempted—completely unfairly but remember this is make-believe—to imagine that she was as wonderful a dominatrix as she seems to have been lawyer, mother, and friend. What she wasn't, one assumes, is someone who might have been dominated into dominating or, for that matter, into being dominated.

The rules are different, however, for sex with prostitutes. A prostitute, no matter how refined or how highly paid, is from the vantage point of her customer the sort of primitive selfobject that Kohut says the small child expects to control as absolutely as an adult expects to control a limb. (Kohut 1971, p. 27). Her satisfaction isn't the concern of her client: she is presumably satisfied the moment she collects her fee—rather like Freud's prescription for psychoanalysts, come to think of it. This suggests that what Spitzer may have needed for the temporarily corrective emotional experience he sought may have been impossible for his wife to provide, because what he may have needed was a self-object he could, in fantasy, absolutely. control. Think of the compliant little boy always striving—perhaps unconsciously sadly and angrily—to do his father's and, doubtless before that, his mother's bidding. The antidote for this may have been a self-object completely antithetical to the accomplished Silda, whom Kohut would have called an "independent center of initiative" (Kohut 1972, p. 363), but identical to Kristen, that is, a self object who would be his to command because his to buy. Indeed, Kristen has said that Spitzer had no interest in getting to know her like some of her other Johns but was instead all business, (Dagostino 2008), so much so that while they had sex he never took off his gartered socks. (Weiss 2008).

By contrast consider Bill Clinton, a man similarly driven by a need to act out sexually and undone by his carelessness. Unlike Spitzer—who wanted ritualized sex from an anonymous stranger whose real name he never knew and who knew him only by a number—Clinton wanted a relationship. He didn't pay Monica Lewinsky, he wooed her, bought her presents and evidently craved her admiration. Indeed, it seems that what he needed from Monica wasn't primitive control, but something akin to what Kohut calls "the gleam in the mother's eye" (Kohut 1971, pp. 116–117). But although Clinton's split-off erotic needs seem more relational than those of Spitzer, and thus perhaps further advanced along a Kohutian developmental line, it isn't clear that the Clintons had a better marriage. We don't know whether Silda Spitzer felt comforted to think the women her husband slept with meant nothing to him or how Hillary felt knowing that Bill thought he was in love with Monica. In any event Bill Clinton seems less split than Eliot Spitzer, less unable to acknowledge his misbehavior. He never pretended to be a puritan and when his affair became public, he didn't resign from office. He fought through an impeachment trial that splashed every nuance of his illicit sex life on the world's front pages as if he'd been born with an immunity to shame.

Given that Eliot Spitzer used prostitutes for at least ten years before being found out, it may be tempting to think that what led to his fall was precisely his becoming Governor. Perhaps not, however, because becoming Governor represented an Oedipal victory so much as it was, to use Paumgarten's term, humbling. And this I suspect had much to do with the fact that Spitzer's abrasive personality—a personality well- suited to the job of prosecuting mobsters, Wall Street cheats and corrupt politicians—didn't work in an office that required him to be comfortable with bedfellows of the political rather than the sexual sort, they didn't want a steamroller so much as someone who could roll with a punch and would be willing to go along to get along, things the uncompromising Spitzer found all but impossible to do. But if he was abrasive, we might think it was to defend against early experiences that left him feeling bruised and damaged because he felt lovable only when he was flattening whoever stood in the way of his father's ambitions. Silda says that she left her law firm to help him campaign because she thought he was too fragile to manage without her. This is a surprising assessment given that fragility is probably the last thing most people think of when they think of Eliot Spitzer. It seems, then, that wounded narcissism, or to put it more familiarly, pride and not guilt is what comes before Eliot Spitzer's fall.

Any psychoanalyst would find it hard not to notice the nearness in age of Kristen and Spitzer's daughters. Kristen was 22 when she was seeing Spitzer, his oldest daughter about 18. Freud would say that Spitzer's unconscious incestuous desires were awakened by living in a household with three teenage girls and, that to keep these impulses at bay, he saw a young prostitute. Kohut might counter that the wounds to Spitzer's narcissism that his trials in office would have brought him every day would have been exacerbated by his exclusion from the intense feminine world of these girls and their mother. However true it may be that no man is a hero to his valet, it is surely truer that no man is a hero to his teenage daughters. The days of father knowing best have long since flown. To Kristen, however, Client Nine was a big shot. And, ironically, although unlike his daughters she had no idea he was in fact the most important man in New York, he was paying her a fortune to make him feel like he was.

I suspect that Silda is right about her husband's emotional fragility. If he were my patient during this second imaginary analysis, I would come to see him as someone subject to depression in the face of narcissistic injuries and/or to overstimulation in the face of triumphs, and who sought to ward off these painful affects by sexualizing his early unmet narcissistic needs in reparative erotic rituals. Treatment for sexual addictions, like that for most behavior disorders, usually follows the lead of twelve-step programs that seek to strengthen the ego's ability to resist temptation by siding with the superego and urging restraint. The problem with such treatments, however, is that they ignore the split-off depression at the heart of sexual acting out and fail to recognize that such errant behavior represents the subject's misbegotten attempt to self-medicate.

Goldberg has taught that cure for these conditions is possible only when the occulted depression is brought into the transference relationship and thus made available for a working through process that can heal the split and make the divided self whole (Goldberg 1999, pp. 103–115).

Spitzer was careless about protecting himself from the dangers to which his expensive and reckless behavior exposed him. because sexualization carries with it an efflorescence of split-off and, thus, unrealistic grandiosity. I doubt that his unconscious intent in spending money lavishly on prostitutes was to fail. Rather it was to defend both his career and his marriage from the vulnerabilities within himself that he knew threatened them. Indeed, he may have thought that by seeing prostitutes, he was protecting his marriage in part by making it impossible for Silda to refuse him and thus locking his potential for rage outside of their bedroom. But as is so often the case with defenses in behavior disorders, the price he had to pay for acting out sexually with Kristen wasn't exacted in the dollars he paid for her services, it was exacted in the blindness that kept him from seeing that what he was doing would eventually destroy him.

Lately, we have been seeing repetitions of such blindness among the rich and powerful everywhere from the automobile industry CEOS who came to Washington in their corporate jets to beg for money, to the Wall Street bankers who paid themselves 18 billion dollars in bonuses out of the TARP (Troubled Asset Recovery Program) money the taxpayers lent them, to John Thaine of Merrill Lynch—(something perhaps of a latter day Thane of Cawdor—you remember, the traitor whose title Duncan awards to Macbeth and of whom it is said that nothing in his life became him like the leaving it). This loathsome Thaine who spent 1.2 million dollars of our money to redecorate his office, most famously on a $35,000 antique commode, perhaps in the infantile certitude that whatever he might deposit there we would consider a treasure. These idiots—as Missouri senator Claire McCaskill has called them—have made everyone from Barack Obama on down ask what in the world they were thinking (Stein 2009). And of course what these scum bag millionaires were thinking is that they deserved everything they took because they were in effect driving under the influence of vertically split-off grandiosity.

Kohut has no name for the Tragic Man (Kohut 1977, pp. 220–248) who opposes Freud's guilt-ridden Oedipus. If we were to give him one we might consider Icarus, the son—in Greek mythology—of the Great Maze-Maker, Daedalus. Daedalus didn't fear his child would destroy him, as did Oedipus's father Laius, but rather that Icarus would destroy himself should he be unable to control the wings he—Daedalus—had given him to soar above all mankind. Daedalus used his art to launch his son into the sky even as Bernard Spitzer used his money to launch his son's quest to become the first Jewish President of the United States. But Icarus became overstimulated and flew too close to the sun which melted his wings and sent him plummeting into the sea. Spitzer became overstimulated and illegally spent five million dollars of his father's money to get elected Attorney General and only narrowly escaped political ruin years before his relation to Kristen brought him down. I think he fell not because he unconsciously feared his father needed him to fail, but rather because he unconsciously understood how much his father needed him to succeed.

REFERENCES

DAGOSTINO, M. (2008). Ex-Call Girl Ashley Dupre: "I'm a normal girl." www.*People.com,* November 19, 2008.

FERMINO, J. (2008). Missus Sacrificed to be Wife and Mom. *The New York Post,* March 11, 2008.

FINEMAN, H. (2008). Notes on a Scandal. *Newsweek*, March 10, 2008.

FISHMAN, S. (2007). The Steamroller in the Swamp: Is Eliot Spitzer Changing Albany? Or is Albany Changing Him? *New York*, July 16, 2007.

FREUD, S. (1916). Those Wrecked by Success. *Standard Edition.* London, Hogarth. 14:303–333, 1957.

GOLDBERG, A. (1995). *The Problem of Perversion.* New Haven: Yale.

——— (1999). *Being of Two Minds.* Hillsdale, The Analytic Press.

KOHUT, H. (1971). *The Analysis of the Self.* New York: International Universities Press.

——— (1972). Thoughts on Narcissism and Narcissistic Rage. *Psychoanalytic Study of the Child* 27: 360–400.

——— (1977). *The Restoration of the Self.* Madison. International Universities Press.

——— (1979), The Two Analyses of Mr Z. *International Journal of Psychoanalysis,* 60:3–27.

NEWMAN, K. (1996). Winnicott Goes To The Movies: The False Self In Ordinary People. *Psychoanalytic Quarterly.* 65:787–807.

PAUMGARTEN, N. (2007). The Humbling of Eliot Spitzer. *The New Yorker.* 12/10/07.

PEARSON, E. AND STANDORA, L. (2009). Madam's Tell-all Book Reveals Eliot Spitzer Scandal Dirt. *www.NewYorkDailyNews.com,* February 6, 2009.

POLLITT, K. (2008). 'John' Q. Public. *The Nation,* March 13, 2008.

ROTH, P. (1969). *Portnoy's Complaint.* New York: Random House.
RUSH, G. & MOLLOY, J. (2009) Eliot Spitzer Choked Her During Sex, Claims High-end Call Girl. *New York Daily News Dot Com.* March 9, 2009.
SCHEIBER, N. (2008). *Eliot Spitzer as Alexander Portnoy.* The New Republic, November 3, 2008.
STANLEY, A. (2008). Mars and Venus Dissect the Spitzer Scandal on the TV Talk Shows. *www.NYTimes*.com, Posted on March 12, 2008.
STEIN, S. (2009). Claire McCaskill Lays Down Law on CEO Compensation www.*HuffingtonPost.com,* January 30, 2009.
THOMAS, E., KLIFF, S., CONANT, E., HOSSENBAL., M, RAMIREZ, J., SMALLEY, S., STONE, D., & TUTTLE, S. (2008). His Dark Journey. *Newsweek,* March 24, 2008.
WEISS, P. (2008). The Affairs of Men: The Trouble with Sex and Marriage. *New York Magazine,* May 18, 2008.
WEISS, M. (2008). Spitzer Redux: Second Prostitute Tells Feds of Ex-Gov's Bedroom Habits. *New York Post,* April 24, 2008.
WHITE, D. (2009). Profile of Eliot Spitzer, Governor of New York posted on www.*about.com,* March 13, 2009.
ZIZAC, S. (2001). *Enjoy Your Symptom.* New York: Rutledge.

Jeffrey Stern
1928 W Grace Street
Chicago, IL 60613–2726
Sternjeffrey@earthlink.net

Richard H. Tuch

CHAPTER 4

Bogus Aims, Unpossessable Objects, Elusive Goals: A Further Contribution to the Psychoanalytic Theory of Greed

Poverty wants much; but avarice, everything.
---PUBLILIUS SYRUS, 1st Century, B.C.

For a host of reasons, greed remains an underdeveloped and underutilized concept in psychoanalytic theory and practice. Greed per se is never offered as a patient's presenting complaint though greed can lead to a chronic sense of dissatisfaction sufficient to drive one to seek treatment. The clinical recognition of greed is further hampered by the fact that many clinicians eschew thinking of their patients as greedy. I suspect this is the result of efforts to protect against inadvertently conveying a negatively charged value judgment about the patient. Empathy for those who act on their greedy impulses proves to be a stretch for some. Judgmental reactions toward those who act greedily may preclude the adoption of a neutral, inquisitive stance needed to further our theoretical understanding of this topic. In addition, our thinking about greed is clouded by difficulties delineating the point at which an inability to feel satisfied, in the face of what appears to be adequate provisions, can reasonably be called greedy. Klein (1975) defines greed as "an impetuous and insatiable craving, exceeding what the subject needs . . ." but how exactly does one measure another's need? How much should be enough?

Greed can be defined as *an inability to ever feel satisfied in spite of sufficient and available supplies that would satisfy most others, leading to an endless search for more and more and more.* Greed is evident when someone perennially pursues a wished-for goal that exceeds what the individual actually needs. While it can be difficult to identify instances when this is the case given that need is relative, greed can be presumed to exist when the continual pursuit of satisfaction fails to bring him or her any closer to the achievement of that goal. No matter how much a greedy individual acquires it never seems to be enough. A constant lack of satisfaction produces a constant, unrelenting pressure that drives the greedy individual toward a goal that ultimately proves unachievable. Greed can be measured, in part, by an individual's continual failure to obtain even a modicum of satisfaction.

In this paper, I will identify three particular aspects of greed and demonstrate how these manifest themselves clinically in the pursuit of bogus aims, attempts to possess and incorporate an object that ultimately proves unpossessable, and an endless search for the unattainable elusive ideal object.. Greed is often the result when an individual misunderstands what it is he or she is actually seeking and mistakenly seeks satisfaction of a "bogus," though tangentially related, desire. This, then, becomes a surrogate for what he actually needs yet can't acknowledge needing. This bogus aim can't possibly satisfy the individual's core, desire and the continuing lack of satisfaction fuels his perennial pursuit of the unattainable atisfaction. Greed also manifests as an attempt to take utter and complete control over one's object, to possess another so as to obliterate any sense of separateness between self and other, Nothing short of complete possession and incorporation will satisfy. Greed is also evident in a pursuit of elusive goals—the search for an ideal object against which no real object can compare. Consider the case of a man who becomes emotionally involved with one woman after another yet can't commit to any of these relationships.Oftentimes this reflects the man's belief that *the* ideal woman does, in fact, exist, leading him on a unrelenting quest to find his dream mate, never realizing all the while that he is waiting for Godot. Though some might chalk this up to a "fear of intimacy" it proves to be a great deal more complex.

GREEDINESS

Strictly speaking, the wish to have it all, and then some, is probably universal. Experiencing compelling needs that produce tensions that seek relief is part of the human condition. The question is how far is an individual willing to go in search of satisfaction. Constitutional factors may play a role in determining one's propensity to act greedily. The strength of one's superego is also a factor that helps determine whether greedy wishes are permitted to become greedy actions. A well-developed superego is likely to inhibit certain individuals from *acting* greedily or *engaging* in outright thievery, even when the wish to get all one can remains an active unconscious fantasy.

Greed can manifest in any number of ways. It can result in the insatiable acquisition of tangible items, such as fortune, or the endless pursuit of such intangibles as fame. It can also manifest as an insatiable thirst for supplies possessed by another who can bestow these supplies as he or she sees fit. (This paper focuses on the enactment of a greedy impulse within the interpersonal sphere). While greed may manifest as a drive to acquire vast amounts of material goods, admirable qualities or attractive traits, it is fair to assume, in most cases, that the goal of ultimately translates into being better positioned to attract more friends and/or lovers. When greedy individuals take a more direct path to acquire supplies possessed by others (i.e., love, attention, admiration, mirroring, etc), it produces a predictable pattern of behaviors. The individual typically lacks the patience required to negotiate with others for a transfer of the goods sought. The sense of vulnerability and powerlessness, along with the anxiety and narcissistic injury—the imagined prospect of being refused and having to do without—oftentimes prove more than the greedy individual can bear. To circumvent the possibility of this emotional calamity, the greedy individual resorts to taking from others, rather than receiving from others. He grabs what he can, ruthlessly pursuing his goals, doing whatever it takes to satisfy his ultimately unquenchable need,. Greed results in a continual striving to acquire more and more in the misguided belief that there is an end in sight.

Psychoanalytic Theories about Greed

The best-known attempt to approach the topic of greed in a theoretically comprehensive fashion was undertaken by Melanie Klein (1975) in her classic work *Envy and Gratitude*, and most psychoanalytic authors who address this subject are quick to cite her work (Riviere 1937; Boris 1986; Kaplan 1991; Waska 1999, 2003; Lamothe 2003). Whereas Freud (1917) believed that greed sprang from anal-erotic wishes, Klein saw it driven by one's oral-aggressive impulses. In her conceptualization of greed, Klein (1975) links deprivation with frustration that, in turn, results in aggression. Such aggression contributes to the fantasy of either the object's retaliatory attack or its passive-aggressive withholding of needed supplies, which furthers the frustration. Taking Klein's thinking a bit further, we can imagine how the frustrated individual might feel the need to rectify matters by taking them into his own hands—by taking what he feels he must have—factoring out the object's willing participation that had previously been required. Such is the nature of interpersonal greed—an imagined tug-of-war between the individual's attempts to procure the needed supplies and the withholding object that steadfastly refuses to provide. Attempting an end run around the object's autonomy in order to ensure one's needs are unquestioningly met isn't so much a matter of entitlement as it is a belief that one's literal psychic survival is at stake.

Klein's explanation of how envy and greed are related furthers our understanding about greed. The infant may project/attribute its hostile, hateful, destructive feelings into the breast, leading to persecutory anxiety. Alternately, the infant may project/attribute its own positive attributes, leading to an idealization of the breast and a concomitant lowering of the infant's sense of value and worth, thus heightening the infant's envy inthe process. If the baby's envious attacks on the breast destroy what is good in the breast, what is left for the baby to internalize from the breast is worthless, at best, if not downright toxic[1]. Since there is no way for a devalued/destroyed breast to nourish, the baby can never feel satisfied no matter how long or how hard it sucks. Accordingly, it remains ravenously hungry in every sense of the word, greedy to the extent it can't ever be satisfied. Klein outlines how greed develops, not only after one has enviously destroyed the breast but also as a preemptive, but ultimately unsuccessful, defense against envy by procuring all of the breast's supplies: "By internalizing the breast so greedily that in the infant's mind it becomes entirely his possession and controlled by him, he feels that all the good that he attributes to it will be his own. This is used to counteract envy. It is the very greed with which this internalization is carried out that contains the germ of failure. . . . By powerful and violent possessiveness, the good object is felt to turn into a destroyed persecutor and the consequences of envy are not sufficiently prevented." (Klein 1975, p. 218).

A Two-Person Psychology Perspective on Greed

Klein makes clear her belief that a sense of deprivation arises not just from internal sources but from external ones as well. Internal (constitutional) factors include: excessive need, an inordinate amount of aggression, low frustration tolerance, etc.. These factors contribute to determining whether provisions prove sufficient to satisfy. As for the external sources of greed, we return to the opening paragraph of this paper. Why not put the full quote in one place at the beginning and refer back to it here? Splitting it up is awkward. (Only half of Klein's (1975) full statement is quoted here. The full statement reads: "Greed is an impetuous and insatiable craving, exceeding what the subject needs *and what the object is able and willing to give*"[2] (p. 18).) In this one sentence Klein simultaneously provides both a one- and a two-person psychology perspective on greed. The first half of the sentence spells out the seemingly limitless nature of a greedy individual's desire regardless of the context or the supplies he has been provided—the one-person psychology perspective. The second half of Klein's statement provides context to the greedy individual's pursuit—the measure of one's need *relative* to what the object is willing to offer. The greedy individual seeks something *from a given other* which that other, due either to lack of desire or ability, fails to provide in full. In such instances, greed approaches a co-constructed/two-person phenomenon in that both parties contribute to its development. This leaves us to wonder whether certain individuals who are not, under normal circumstances, innately greedy might be enticed to become so under conditions that stimulate a powerful need yet leave that need unfulfilled. Sadistic teasing comes to mind, but there may be many other conditions that operate along such lines.

BOGUS AIMS: GREED AND THE EROTICIZED TRANSFERENCE

For some patients the conditions of psychoanalytic treatment—the psychoanalyst's attunement to subtle affect, capacity for empathic understanding, tenderness, kindness and undivided attention—runs the risk of stimulating hope that the analyst will provide much more than he/she actually plans to deliver. Some patients develop erotic fantasies about the analyst and a few go on to consider these fantasies a real possibility. Half-hoping to effect such an outcome, these patients press on in the belief that the analyst will eventually succumb to their seduction so long as the patient waits patiently and plays his or her cards right.

This brings us to a topic not typically associated with greed—that of "the eroticized transference" (Rappaport, 1956; Person, 1985)—"an intense, vivid, irrational, erotic preoccupation with the analyst, characterized by overt, seemingly egosyntonic demands for love and sexual fulfillment from the analyst" (Blum 1973, p. 63).—which is distinguishable from the more commonly encountered forms of transference love ("erotic transference") evident when "a woman patient shows by unmistakable indications, or openly declares, that she has fallen in love, as any other mortal woman might, with the doctor who is analyzing her"

(Freud 1915 p. 159). While Blum considers the eroticized transferences nothing more than an extreme form of erotic transference, not all agree (Bibring 1936; Rappaport 1956; Person 1985; Trop 1988), arguing the two differ in important ways even though they share surface similarities—the patient's proclamation of love for the analyst.

Though Freud never used the term "eroticized transference" he did identify a group of woman who we would now consider to manifest an eroticized transference: "women of elemental passionateness who tolerate no surrogates. They are children of nature who refuse to accept the psychical in place of the material, who, in the poet's words, are accessible only to 'the logic of soup, with dumplings for arguments'. With such people one has the choice between returning their love or else bringing down upon oneself the full enmity of a woman scorned. In neither case can one safeguard the interests of the treatment" (Freud 1915, pp. 165–166).

As Freud notes, cases of eroticized transference typically present a formidable challenge to the analyst's continued ability to operate analytically. The most extreme cases of eroticized transference, in contrast with more garden-variety types of transference love, involve patients who refuse to consider the possibility that their professed love represents more than it appears to represent at first glance. Swept up and lost in their feelings of love, these patients often refuse to "play by the psychoanalytic rules." While they may humor the analyst by acting as if they have adopted the spirit of analysis, it eventually becomes clear this is little more than a ruse—a way of buying time so that they can press their love agenda. Some of these patients turn away from recognizing the "as if" aspect of the transference, others prove utterly blind to this perspective. Convinced by the compelling reality of their feelings, these patients dismiss attempts to clarify or interpret them. They consider such attempts ludicrous—a manifestation of the analyst's laughable search for underlying meanings beneath obvious and uncomplicated circumstances.

One unfortunate result of such enacted eroticized transferences is that they can derail the entire psychoanalytic venture. "The specialness of the eroticized transference," Wilson (1984) notes, "is in its rendering ineffectual the ordinary analytic modalities. . . with this rejection of verbalization, the refusal of shared signifiers and the demand for another type of sharing, the analyst's purpose, his raison d'être, his primary tool for analytic work is forfeited" (p. 307).

So how does greed fit in here? The clinical behavior of patients seized by the most extreme forms of eroticized transference makes it abundantly clear that they are hell bent on getting what they want, and all that they want, regardless of the analyst's plans or wishes. Such patients become singularly focused on this task and work to wear the analyst down, to chip away at his resistance, until he or she tires, caves in, and submits to the patient's demands. Though the analyst struggles mightily to maintain the frame, the patient is forever challenging limits in ways that leave the analyst no feasible option but to set and enforce strict limits, which runs counter to how analysts like to operate.

In many instances, pressing for the enactment of love is but one of the many ways such patients push the envelope in an effort to break through established and inherent barriers. Their wishes extend far beyond merely sleeping with the analyst and include dismantling each and every inherent boundary that separates the two. Patients in the throes of an eroticized transference bitterly protest and refuse the task of reconciling themselves to a piece of unyielding reality—the fact that they cannot take utter and sole possession of the analyst. The intense pre-oedipal, narcissistic anxieties experienced by these patients drives them onward, lending greed its unrelenting quality. The successful seduction of the analyst promises to lend credence to the patient's omnipotent fantasy of being the "irresistible seductress" (Blum 1973; Coen 1981). For these patients, nothing short of sexual intercourse with the analyst can establish their specialness since they fantasize that they'd be the first and only patient to succeed in this fashion (Blum 1973; Trop 1988). They think that such an outcome might even be sufficiently transformational as to render further treatment unnecessary.

Beyond this particular aim, some patients may seek "to excite and enslave [their] devalued partner" (Blum 1973, p. 65) in an act of retribution and triumphant reversal for the same having been done to them in childhood. The eroticized transference also serves to gain and exert complete control over the analyst in an effort to circumvent the problems inherent in depending upon others. This maneuver enables the patient to avoid having to come to terms with the analyst's independent and relatively autonomous existence—someone upon whom the patient must rely to get his or her needs met. This runs counter to the patient's preferred fantasy that satisfaction is something that is completely under his/her control—something he or she can make happen at will.

EROTICIZED TRANSFERENCE REFLECTING GREED

Greed sometimes appears in the consultation room in the form of an intractable eroticized transference, as illustrated by the following clinical example. Mrs. B., a 27-year-old married woman born in the Middle-East, was referred to Dr. P. for marital counseling. Mrs. B. harbored anger and resentment toward her husband and was unsure whether she wanted to stay married. The patient had long flirted with older men who were in positions of authority and she had gone on to marry a Middle-Eastern man 25 years her senior whom she'd met on a visit home. The patient married her husband after having known him for only a short time. When she asked herself why she had acted so hastily, she rationalized that it was her way of helping support her mother who, having been left years before by the father, was barely making ends meet. Her fiancé promised to purchase a condominium for the mother, which he did once the couple had wed.

During her latency the patient's parents divorced. After the divorce the patient carried on a distant relationship with her father, a man who disgusted her, who seemed disinterested in her, and who failed to provide financial support for she and her family. The patient's relationship with her mother was characterized by anxious-dependent attachment. She slept in her mother's bed well into adolescence.

Aside from the trouble she had controlling her impulses, the patient suffered from low self-esteem and had trouble respecting boundaries. She had pursued her husband's brother, a married man who showered her with attention and affection. She considered him to be everything her husband was not—educated, charming, ambitious and financially stable—and the two carried on an affair that was still active at the time she entered analysis.

There were other ways the patient challenged established boundaries and limits. Growing up under the strict rules for women in the Middle East left Mrs. B. envious of the freedom afforded boys. At one point she cut her hair quite short thus changing her appearance to that of a boy so as to evade school rules that prohibited girls from being on the playground with boys. In her mid-teens the patient began to flirt with men in their fifties and took to hanging around a particular storeowner's shop until she was told her obvious interest in him was inappropriate. When she turned eighteen, she carried on a clandestine two-year relationship with a man in his mid-thirties who she only later learned was married and had two children, another source (but not the original) of her intense anger at men in general. Mrs. B. was generally distrustful and disdainful of men who she regarded as weak: "All you have to do is flirt with them or offer them sex. It doesn't matter who they are. All the men I work with flirt with me."

Not long after the patient and her husband began couple's therapy, the therapist decided that she could accomplish more were Mrs. B. to be seen in individual psychotherapy. Several months after beginning psychoanalytically-oriented psychotherapy, the psychologist, a candidate in psychoanalytic training, converted her treatment to a control case. That candidate came to me for supervision and the information presented in this paper was gleaned from his presentation of the case over the course of a year. Treatment was conducted at a frequency of four times weekly, with the patient alternating between being on and off the couch.

Though both patient and analyst were fluent in English, they hailed from the same country and the treatment was conducted in their native tongue. I suspect this further heightened the intimacy experienced by the patient given that everyone in the adjoining offices of the psychotherapy suite was speaking English. Those fluent in a second language sometimes shift into speaking that language when they want to hide what they are saying from others.

Shortly after the analysis began it became clear that this was far from an ideal control case. The patient professed her love for the analyst, declaring that she *had* to have him. She claimed to know for certain that he, too, would be happy were they to be together. She told him she had never before met a man like him and praised him to the hilt. She was comfortable with him and felt she could speak openly with him as she had with no other person in her life. Being with the analyst romantically, the patient argued, would obviate the need for treatment since she would then have everything her heart desired.

Sometimes Mrs. B. expressed gratitude that the analyst hadn't fallen for her seductions as had all the other men, but the next moment she was again wholeheartedly pursing her explicit and stated goal of making the analyst hers and hers alone. She considered her love for the analyst reality-based so it only seemed natural to her that they become romantically involved. This goal seemed reasonable, the patient added, so there was no need to analyze these wishes. Certainly she would feel no different had the two met under other circumstance. In fact, she reminded the analyst, they had met sometime before treatment began, even though the analyst hadn't remembered the event. The analyst wracked his brain but couldn't recall the incident, and it was weeks before the patient admitted she had made the whole story up in order to undermine the analyst's position that her love was transferential in nature. Lying in this way illustrates the lengths to which this patient would go to get what she wanted, seemingly indifferent to the way in which her actions perverted her relationship with the analyst and undermined the entire psychoanalytic venture.

Mrs. B. thought about her analyst night and day. She would often wake in the morning feeling his body next to hers only to realize, with great disappointment, that it was not he but her husband. She frequently would leave urgent voicemail messages that made it sound as if she was in desperate need that necessitated a timely response. The analyst accepted the patient's portrayed need at face value leading him to call her back on a regular basis—a practice that continued until supervision helped the candidate extricate himself from these enactments as he came to appreciate her portrayal of urgency as just that, a portrayal.

The patient engaged in every sort of enactment. She came to sessions dressed provocatively, sometimes stopping home after work to slip into something more enticing. She would force herself on the analyst physically, leading with her breasts—a maneuver that had him literally struggling to keep her at arms length. Unfortunately, her scheduled session tended to be the candidate's last session of the day making it easier for her to refuse to leave, knowing the analyst had no one else to see that day other than his wife and children who, she surmised, were waiting for him at home. The patient's refusal to leave sometimes extended the session for upwards of thirty minutes. Oft times, when the analyst was able to move her out of the consulting room at the session's end, the patient would follow him to his car, and once stole his car keys away from him just as she had grabbed the T.V. remote from her father when she was young, hiding it where he could not reach it. It would have been easy to interpret the patient's behavior strictly in oedipal terms, for example, as a wish to keep him from going home to his wife, were it not for the fact that most of the patient's material was decidedly pre-oedipal and narcissistic in nature.

There was no end to the pleasure the patient seemed to derive from playing a cat and mouse game with her "captured prey". Sometimes she would position herself on the floor, gradually inching her way toward the analyst as the session progressed so that she could then pounce on to his lap before he'd have a chance to fend her off. If one were to paint a picture that captured the condition of the analysis it would be that of a patient, full of glee and triumphant excitement, madly chasing the analyst about the room with the analyst sweating profusely with a lost, panicked look on his face.

Try as he might to set rules and enforce limits, it proved nearly impossible to rein the patient in and gain a reasonable semblance of control. During the analysis no true therapeutic alliance was ever formed. It became increasingly obvious that the patient had no intention whatsoever of engaging in an exploration of her feelings. Efforts to interpret the underlying pre-oedipal needs that masqueraded as adult sexual feelings fell on deaf ears. The patient was having none of it. Aside from her inability, or refusal, to work analytically, the patient's behavior taxed her analyst's patience. At times her idealization of him and her proclamations of love proved narcissistically gratifying in that they left the analyst feeling loved, admired, and desired. Such is the nature of seduction. At other times the analyst experienced such a degree of confusion, fear, impotence, anger and frustration that he found it impossible to sufficiently contain these feelings so as to process and re-present these feelings in a form the patient could use. The analyst often felt out of control, unsure of how to bring the situation back under control so that he could get back to the task of conducting an analysis. Sometimes the patient's outrageousness behavior even made it hard for him to think, leading him to entertain the idea of transferring the case, figuring Mrs. B.'s eroticized transference could not be handled in any other way.

The case of Mrs. B. is very much like another I had reported in the literature (Tuch 2007), a case of a gay patient who developed an eroticized transference to me. Mr. A. would intermittently plant kisses on my lips and trespass on my body by touching me whenever and wherever he chose. Just as Mrs. B. made her analyst feel, Mr. A. also caused me to feel as if I were being chased about the room. His outrageous behavior knew no bounds: "Mr. A. would rail against every conceivable boundary. He had strong reactions to the beginning and the end of every session, as well as to anything that demarcated my separate life, be it evidence of my separate subjectivity, my private thoughts, or my life away from him. Limits were a particular problem. The time-limited nature of our sessions was something he particularly couldn't stand, and any sign that I had been looking in the clock's direction produced rage and charges that I didn't love him and couldn't wait to be rid of him. He often turned my clocks around so that I wouldn't know when the session was drawing to an end. Sessions typically began in the waiting room. On the way in, Mr. A. would rub up against me the way a cat would its owner, pressing up against me long enough to leave a scent of his cologne, ensuring that I'd become similarly scented—a sort of olfactory forget-me-not that would linger for hours. It was as if the patient had marked his territory . . . Once in the room, Mr. A. took the liberty of sitting anywhere he chose, including at my desk where he would rifle through my papers. He enjoyed my obvious annoyance, which left me feeling outraged and on edge, unable to consistently maintain an ability to think analytically." (Tuch 2007, p. 104)

Unlike Mr. A., who finally settled down so that we could do some work, Mrs. B.'s analysis ultimately had to be interrupted. Summing the situation up, the analyst wrote: "I tried to help Mrs. B. understand and bring into her conscious awareness the importance of the deeply hidden meaning of her erotic and idealized transference toward me . . . however, the patient continuously and insistently claimed that her love for me was real and not infantile in nature. She could not see the compulsive and obsessional characteristic of her transference love and resisted any interpretative attempts on my part. She was too dedicated to action regardless of my efforts to help her understand the meaning of her actions. She refused to have any regard for reality, and was blind to the consequences of her feelings, thoughts and fantasies. She also remained blind to the 'as if' quality of her feelings toward me and insisted on them as being real and normal."

As the quotation that headlines this paper notes, avarice wants everything, and that precisely defines what Mrs. B. and Mr. A. desired. Though each of these patients framed their desires in terms of adult erotic desire, every aspect of their ways of relating to the analyst belied a deeper and broader interest in gaining complete control. Their goal was to make him theirs or, more precisely, to make themselves one and the same as the analyst—to pervert the relationship by attempting to obliterate differences between the two (Chasseguet-Smirgel 1984) so as to not have to experience needs that could only be satisfied by an autonomous other. This is what defined these patients' greed—their insatiable desire to have everything, to own the analyst so that they would never have to experience a sense of unbearable separateness and, with it, a potentially insatiable need. Just as she had been anxiously dependent upon her mother, Mrs. B. now transferred these needs to her analyst, though she dressed them up in adult clothing and sold herself, and her analyst, on the notion that she was burning with sexual desire that could only be quenched in bed. The same was true of Mr. A., who railed against anything that established a difference between him and me.

Eroticized Transferences Not Reflecting Greed

Before moving on to a consideration of other clinical manifestations of greed, it should be noted that not all cases of eroticized transference prove as difficult to treat, and not all represent instances of greed. Blum describes two cases (1971, 1973): the first—a single woman whose initial eroticized transference ultimately blossomed into an Oedipal-based transference neurosis—and the second—a young married woman who presented with depression, frigidity and pseudonymphomania who came to think of the analysis as a clandestine affair. This later patient became flirtatious and seductive with her analyst, ultimately announcing her attraction and proposing the two have sexual relations right then and there on the analyst's couch. Sex with the analyst would not only be beautiful, the patient declared, but therapeutic in that it would dislodge the analyst from his "aloof" analytic stance. In addition, it would confirm that she was his favorite patient and thus help bolster her low self-esteem and intense feelings of narcissistic vulnerability. Blum notes this patient was "more anxious and entreating than insatiable" (p. 65), in distinction to Mrs. B. and Mr. A., and her eroticized transference, like that of the first patient Blum described, also proved treatable as a transference neurosis.

Trop (1988) presents clinical material about a patient who is similar to Blum's second patient. In this he demonstrates how an eroticized transference can sometime develop as a result of a patient's failed attempt to elicit mirroring from the analyst in response to the exhibition of something other than the patient's sexuality. "Self-esteem in these patients," writes Trop, "is defensively structured around a capacity to engender sexual excitement in another person [when] . . . self-object longings for mirroring are eroticized" (p. 269). He describes how the patient "wanted to feel special and unique" Her behavior was accompanied by a feeling of desperation. She felt that if she could have sex with her analyst she would feel her sense of specialness confirmed by him. She assumed that the therapist had never had sexual relations with any of his patients and that she would be the very first, and only, patient he'd ever desired in this way. It seemed clear she had an intense feeling that she would somehow be permanently transformed by the experience. She had fantasies of watching him becoming excited with her, and felt that he would find her to be unique and unusual in her ability to please him. Although she understood that this was not his role, she felt intensely that it would be the right thing for both of them" (pp. 272–273).

Looking for Love in all the Wrong Places

The eroticized transference is widely understood to be a masquerade. Though the patient portrays what looks very much like adult genital sexuality, it is anything but. Professed interest in becoming sexually involved with the analyst hides the patient's underlying infantile desires—to be rocked, feed and mirrored by a mommy. This defense proves necessary because the patient experiences unbearable feelings of vulnerability and powerlessness in the face of his or her oral dependent needs—needs the patient feels can't be left to chance or maternal fancy to be satisfied. Thinking these needs may go unmet is more than the patient feels he or she can bear. In order to cope, the patient disguises these yearnings as adult sexual desire which places her on equal footing with the analyst, who has adult sexual desires of his own that the patient feels in a position to satisfy.

Taking it a step further, the prospect of successfully seducing the analyst promises to turn the table by making *the analyst* dependent upon *the patient*, thus reversing the patient's childhood circumstances. This hoped for result would reinforce the patient's omnipotent fantasies and contribute to the manic denial of his or her core neediness. By this maneuver, the patient gains illusory control over the source of his/her satisfaction, thus solving the central problem of dependency. Though the defense may seem airtight, the oral demanding nature of the sexual advances—which the patient would like to believe is nothing more than a measure of the strength of his or her libido—is a tip off about the true nature of the patient's needs.

The elements of greed outlined earlier are all evident in the clinical presentation of the eroticized transference. An attempt to get core needs met through the satisfaction of "bogus" needs is one of the root causes of greed. In these cases of eroticized transference, the sexualization of oral-dependent needs caused these patients to seek satisfaction of needs different from the ones that were most pressing. Attempts to take complete control over the object is another manifestation of greed that is quite evident in the clinical presentation of the eroticized transference. The presence of this dynamic may be the factor that distinguishes cases that are analyzable from those that are not. Idealization of the analyst—believing him/her to be the embodiment of the fantasized ideal object—is the final factor that drives such patients to feel they must make the analyst their own. Only he/she—the ideal object—is capable of satisfying the individual's deepest needs.

THE PURSUIT OF "BOGUS" NEEDS

Eric Carle's (1969) much-acclaimed and widely-read children's picture book, *The Very Hungry* Caterpillar, is the tale an insatiable caterpillar who cannot be satisfied no matter how much he eats. Day after day the hungry caterpillar eats his ways through ever increasing quantities of fruits: an apple on Monday, two pears on Tuesday, three plums on Wednesday, etc. No matter how much the caterpillar eats nothing seems to hit the spot, leaving him utterly unsatisfied. By the time Saturday rolls around, hunger drives the caterpillar into a feeding frenzy during which he samples ten different foods and ends up with a stomachache. On Sunday the caterpillar "ate through one nice green leaf, and after that he felt better." Finally satiated, he builds himself a cocoon and emerges, two weeks later, transformed into a beautiful butterfly. The moral to the story is: *trying to satisfy a need by acquiring what one convinces oneself is an equivalent provision won't produce satisfaction; the frustration will persist unabated so long as the search continues down the same path.* Such a self-evident idea would seem to go without saying until one looks around and sees how many people live their lives in ways that contradict this very principle. Greed often arises when the goal pursued differs from the one unconsciously desired.

The eroticized transference is a specific and extreme example of seeking satisfaction through the pursuit of what ultimately proves to be a bogus need that is used to substitute for what an individual primarily needs. There are other less extreme examples where the pursuit of a particular satisfaction fails to alleviate the underlying need. In such instances, awareness of the true nature of one's core needs becomes lost in the process of pursuing the bogus needs. Take, for example, married men who claim to pursue extramarital affairs in search of sexual satisfaction that can't be had sleeping with just one woman. Sexual frustration can account for some, but not all, of these affairs. Often times men are primarily driven by the desire to be desired—by the narcissistic need to conduct a metaphoric survey aimed at re-establishing their sense of attractiveness when it is on the wane. While libidinal desire and needs for mirroring seem easily distinguishable, it sometimes is difficult to disentangle one from the other. Male pride makes many men bristle at the suggestions that there are times when a woman's evident interest and willingness to have sex proves even more satisfying than intercourse itself, a notion some would consider patently ludicrous. However, just like the patient who sexualizes her *oral-dependent needs* resulting in the creation of an eroticized transference, men sometimes sexualize their *narcissistic needs*, which become obscured by the "compelling" argument that men can't seriously be expected to submit to the unnatural and unreasonable societal restriction of monogamy. This isn't to say these men aren't seeking sexual satisfaction, it is only to note the importance of other more pressing needs that often go unacknowledged (Tuch 2000).

Lacan (1977) goes a step further by suggesting that it is impossible to directly satisfy certain core human desires resulting in an inevitable search to satisfy surrogate needs leaving the individual far from satisfied. He argues that human desire ultimately reduces to the desire to be desired. He locates the development of desire in the "mirror stage" of infancy. It is then that the mother forms an imago of whom she imagines the infant to be—which more or less recognizes and incorporates some, but not all, of the infant's innate features. But even when the mother's image of the infant isn't far off the mark, it invariably falls short of completely identifying the infant's core subjectivity—who it experiences itself to be. Lacan argues that the infant identifies with what he or she sees mirrored in the mother's gaze—*her* version of the infant, which the infant then confuses with its own true, subjective self. Thereafter, and forever more, lying behind the ego that seeks to be found is the subjective self that can never entirely be known. The unquenchable thirst to be recognized and desired sets one in perennial pursuit of what ultimately proves an elusive goal—the quest to be *recognized as a subject* distinct from the fantasy-based construct of who the other wishes us into being in their mind's eye—the other's *use of us as an object.*[3] As a result, chasing after another's desire becomes an embedded aspect of ever individuals' desire—searching to discover and embody what it is the other finds desirable. But since one can never be entirely known, the object that ends up being desired is never wholly identical to the human who seeks to be desired.

Unable to satisfy the wish to be thoroughly recognized or truly desired by another for who one experiences oneself to be, humans often redirect themselves toward tangible aims that are within reach. In this fashion, the pursuit of sexual satisfaction, driven by aims of its own, may also serve as proxy for the individual's sexualized wish to be recognized and desired. For this reason, striving to attain a modicum of sexual pleasure often fails to satisfy the core need, leaving much to be desired.

PURSUIT OF ELUSIVE IDEAL OBJECT

Having explored two of the manifestations of greed—the pursuit of bogus aims and the attempt to take complete possession of the object—we now turn our attention to a final factor that further contributes to the genesis of greed: a pursuit of the elusive ideal object—the all-satisfying breast, the incomparable mate, the perfect occupation, etc. Searching for the ideal object keeps one in perpetual motion considering and discarding one potential candidate after another in a mad forage—a gluttonous sampling of the available possibilities none of which seems to measure up to some fantasized ideal that, alone, is capable of satisfying. "There *has* to be more and better options[4]", complains the greedy individual, "this can't possibly be the field from which I am expected to choose." Desperately seeking the "eureka" moment drives the greedy individual onward in search for the fulfillment of his or her dearest fantasy—proof that the ideal object does, indeed, exist so long as one waits patiently, hopes blindly, and steadfastly refuses to settle for anything less.

What is required of an object for it to qualify as ideal? What constitutes the perfect breast? From the standpoint of infantile needs, the ideal object is, first and foremost, a part object (1) that exists for the sole purpose of satisfying one's every wish and need, (2) is wholeheartedly dedicated to that task, and (3) has the wherewithal to supply endlessly without becoming depleted. The ideal object permits no competitors to challenge one's absolute claim on the entirety of the object's supplies, and never allows its autonomous existence, separate subjectivity or personal needs to impinge in ways that might cause the greedy individual guilt for requiring the object to do without. Naturally, the perfect object is a fantasy, though it may well build upon cherished memories when the mother seemed, if only for a moment, to be the endlessly giving and utterly selfless individual the infant wished her to be.

The ideal object is the perfect servant, as conceptualized in Robert Altman's 2001 film *Gosford Park*, a movie that explores the relationships between members of the privileged class who converge on an English manor with their respective servants in tow. One of the servants describes to another what constitutes a perfect servant: one who anticipates the master's needs even before the master realizes he has such needs, then caters to them seamlessly and dutifully. The perfect object rescues the individual from having to experience the tension that necessarily accompanies an emerging need. The master is saved not only from such discomfort, but also from the energy required to conceptualize and articulate what it is he or she needs. He needn't lift a finger nor have a care about his needs going unmet. Banish the thought! The perfect object is, after all, a mind reader. The metaphor of merger seems to capture this experience amply. Such a condition protects one from having to come face to face with the reality of one's separateness with the attendant realization that one is oftentimes at the mercy of others to get one's needs met. In the consulting room, the patient expects to receive perfectly attuned empathic understanding as well as accurate discernment and a continuous gratification of self-object and/or oral-dependent needs. Even in treatment—particularly in treatment—one's hopes to encounter the ideal object will inevitably come to grief, the working through of which some consider to be the central task of treatment.

Another attribute required of the perfect object is illustrated in Shel Silverstein's *The Giving Tree*—a children's tale about the relationship between a mother-tree and a young boy. As the boy grows into adulthood, he never outgrows his use of the tree as a part object to provide for his every need. First, the boy consumes the tree's fruit and plays in its branches. Once an adult, he asks for the tree's trunk which he then turns into lumber to build a boat. By the end of the tale the tree, having acquiesced to each and every one of the boy's requests, has been reduced to a mere stump—whittled away by the man-boy's greedy demands. Even then, the tree stump is happy to have something it can still offer the now-aged man-boy—a place upon which to sit., The selfish and destructive effect of greed is the moral of the story for most though, surprisingly, some have actually taken the tale to be one of admirable, selfless giving. Go figure! As the tree is consumed by the man-boy's needs it only once expresses regret at its fate. This expression of its own feelings reveals it is flawed as an ideal object. Not only does the tree think about its own sacrifice, it also fails to live up to expectation as an ideal object in that it becomes depleted in the process of giving and cannot be relied upon to provide endlessly for the man-boy's needs. The ideal object cannot be either depleted or destroyed in the process of being consumed greedily. That outcome is seen as a betrayal of the perfect object's supposed promise to "be there" forever forever and ever. Such is the myth of unconditional love.

The perfect object must not only lack discernible needs of its own but also have no other masters who might interfere with its being available to attend to its sole master's every wish and whim. Having to wait and watch while the object tends to the needs of another replicates experiences one had with siblings. This can lead to feelings of dependency, frustration, impatience, impotence, jealousy, disappointment, loss, rage and narcissistic injury. These feelings can quickly and efficiently be avoided so long as the perfect object has only one master .

John Fowles' (1997) novel *The Collector* (1963) illustrates the enactment of such a fantasy. A young woman is imprisoned by a man in the basement of his house so that she will always be available to satisfy his needs. Here, greed is demonstrated in the monopolization of resources. The imprisoned woman in Fowles' tale ultimately fails to live up to expectation as the ideal object. She falls ill, and her need to be taken to the hospital runs counter to his need to keep her under lock and key. Thus, she dies, robbing the man of further gratification of his fantasy. Like the man-boy's destructive consumption of the giving tree, this man's greedy possession of this woman ultimately destroys her. The true perfect object, by definition, can never be destroyed no matter how compromised its own sources of life-sustaining nourishment.

Although the greedy individual might intellectually acknowledge the ideal object to be nothing more than a fantasy, his actions run counter to this acknowledgment given his inability to accept provisions others would consider ample. The greedy individual insists he is not being unreasonable when he refuses to "settle," he is just remaining true to his ideals by refusing to give up on his dreams. He holds out hope that the ideal object actually exists, one that would not only satisfy his every wish but would prove worthy of him. In this last statement, we see the greedy individual not only seeking satisfaction of his oral-dependent needs but of his narcissistic needs as well.

The process just described takes place largely on an unconscious level. The individual compares prospective candidates against the fantasized ideal object and concludes, time and again, that this one *also* falls short just as had all the rest that came before. The most obvious example of such thinking is seen in single men who believe themselves to be seriously dating yet, upon further consideration, seem to be doing anything but. Such men become quite interested in a potential mate who they claim they would consider marrying *if only it weren't for X*. The man declares a deep affection for this woman, claiming he can't imagine living without her. However, when he takes inventory of her strengths and weaknesses he comes up with a big "but"—the deal breaker. One woman is a spendthrift, the next is overly frugal; this one is too passive and dependent, the last one had been too independent, etc. Each of these highlighted objections becomes an impossible impediment. Settling down would be nothing more than settling, and that is the last thing the man plans to do. While such thinking is often seen as a man's defense against fears of intimacy, dependency, and commitment, they can also reflect the man's practice of comparing each woman to an unconscious ideal object against which no woman can compare. Greed knows not of the good enough object, leading to the greedy man's failure to ever feel satisfied enough to commit to a long-term relationship.

CONCLUDING REMARKS

Greed is easiest to recognize when an individual has an insatiable desire to acquire an excess of either material or intangible goods. Aside from this obvious manifestation of greed there are other, more obscure ways in which greed may appear, particularly interpersonal greed. In this paper I have examined clinical material that, upon first glance, wouldn't immediately bring greed to mind. The greedy nature of excessive acquisitiveness is far more obvious to most than the covert greediness of an eroticized transference or that of a man who discards a series of love prospects because none lives up to his picture of the ideal mate. When one recognizes how a chronic sense of dissatisfaction can arise from the combined effect of a person's pursuit of bogus aims, his attempts to take complete possession of his object, and his unrelenting pursuit of the ideal object—it becomes apparent how often greed may go unrecognized and underappreciated.

Bulimia is yet another clinical example of greed in action. Seeing bulimia as a form of greed gives us a somewhat different perspective on the condition—an insatiable hunger that drives a person to acts of utter gluttony. Consider the following dynamics: Idealization of the object is, by nature, self-depleting to the extent one loses a sense of one's own value/goodness in the process of projecting or attributing it to another[5]. The resulting lack of a sense of internal value/goodness (having been lost in the projection/attribution) creates, in turn, an awesome hunger. This generates a need to fill the created void by re-internalizing aspects of the now ideal-seeming object. The individual feels he cannot possibly do without these supplies. He or she feels they must get at them no matter what—it is a matter of psychic life or death. Unfettered access to the object's supplies cannot be left to chance. Accordingly, the psychically starved individual must take matters into his or her own hands and get at these life-sustaining supplies in a way that gets around the variability of the object's willingness to supply them.

A solution comes to the bulimic's mind at this point. Through symbolic equation—a process by which the symbol and the symbolized become synonymous—*food quite literally becomes the nurturing object.* Through the use of disavowal, food becomes a fetish—a stand-in for the idealized breast, which can be possessed and is accordingly always available to satisfy. In bulimia *the act of eating* and *the act of being fed* become delinked in much the same way that greed involves *taking* rather than *being given to*, factoring out the object's autonomy in the process. As food had once been associated with mother it now becomes the same as mother, a clever solution to the problem of being at mother's mercy. The greedy urge to take complete possession of the idealized mother, which threatens the mother's destruction and, in turn, can emotionally starve the child, becomes transferred on to a different playing field. Food as a source of psychic, as well as bodily, nourishment can now come under the hungry child's complete possession and control. The child need no longer rely on the whim of the breast to provide.

In the end, however, this solution is flawed. One feels ravenously hungry but can't get enough of what one thinks should sate the hunger. No matter how much one eats it never hits the spot, much like the very hungry caterpillar. The ravenous orality that derives, in part, from the idealization of the object can't possibly be satisfied by dispensing with the object—substituting self-acquirable food in place of the object—the autonomous breast. The momentary satisfaction that comes from engaging in what amounts to hallucinatory wish fulfillment lasts only so long. In the end, the infant awakens to the realization that the imagined breast is illusory and can't hope to satisfy in quite the same way that mother's milk can. So too, food itself can't hope to satisfy if one is actually hungering *to be fed by another*. Long ago, Spitz (1945) established that being fed, in the complete sense of the term, is not the same as being provided with food. Infants who were nourished only with food failed to thrive. Feeding had to be part-and-parcel of an emotional experience with a consistent, reliable, loving other.

Most likely, there are innumerable roots to greed. Although this paper discusses certain aspects of greed, it should not be considered a thorough exploration of the subject. Sometimes greed is the result of the chronic lack of satisfaction that inevitably results when one perennially seeks out that which cannot and will not satisfy. In this case, hunger continues unabated leading to the continuous desperate pursuit of bogus aims, unpossessable objects and elusive goals. Sometimes one grows older, yet fails to outgrow the need to be satisfied in ways only appropriate to infancy. In these cases also, the needs will never be fulfilled satisfactory.

The danger is in thinking of greed in a moral sense—that a greedy individual is utterly unreasonable in that he or she wants more than life can reasonably provide, more than what the rest of us have to settle for and accept. Lack of empathy leads to thinking that greed cannot be treated psychodynamically. To the extent we disown greed within ourselves, we end up scapegoating others who we perceive as greedy. Rescuing those wracked with greed requires we find ways to make their plight something with which we can empathize. If this paper has contributed to that goal, it has accomplished its mission.

REFERENCES

BIBRING, G. (1936). A contribution to the subject of transference resistance, *Internatinoal Journal of Psycho-Analysis* 17:181–189.

BLUM, H. (1971). *Transference and structure. In The Unconscious Today.* Ed. M. Kanzer. New York: International University Press, pp. 177–195

——— (1973). The Concept of Erotized Transference.. *Journal of the American Psychoanalytic Association* 21:61–76

BORIS, H. (1986). The "Other" Breast—Greed, Envy, Spite and Revenge. *Contemporary Psychoanalysis.* 22: 45–59

CARLE, E. (1969). *The Very Hungry Caterpillar.* New York, NY: Philomel (Penguin Group USA)

CHASSEGUET-SMIRGEL, J. (1984). *Creativity and Perversion.* London: Free Ass. Books.

COEN, S. (1981). Sexualization as a Predominant Mode of Defense. *Journal of the American Psychoanalytic Association* 29:893–920.

FOWLES, J. (1997). The Collector. Back Bay Books (Div of Little, Brown).

FREUD, S. (1915). Observations on transference-love *Standard Edition* 12:158–171.

——— (1917). On the transformation of instinct as exemplified in anal-eroticism. *Standard Edition* 17:127–133.

KAPLAN, H. (1991). Greed: A Psychoanalytic Perspective. *Psychoanalytic*

Review 78(4):505–523.

KLEIN, M. (1975). *Envy and gratitude In Envy and Gratitude and Other Works 1946–1963*. London: Hogarth, 1975 pp. 176–235.

LACAN, J. (1977), Écrits. A Selection, trans. A. Sheridan. New York: Norton.

LAMOTHE, R. (2003). Poor Ebenezer: Avarice as Corruption of the Erotic and Search for a Transformative Object. *Psychoanalytic Review* 90:(1) 23–43

PERSON, E.S. (1985). The Erotic Transference in Women and in Men: Differences and Consequences. *Journal of the American Academy of Psychoanalysis* 13:159–8

RAPPAPORT, E. (1956). the Management of an Erotized Transference, *Psychoanalytic Quarterly* 25:515–529.

RIVIERE, J. (1937). Hate, Greed and Aggression, in: *Love, Hate and Reparation* ed. M. Klein. & J. Riviere. London: Hogarth Press, pp. 3–53

SILVERSTEIN S. (1964). *The Giving Tree.* New York: NY: Harpers Collins

SPITZ, R. (1945) Hospitalism: An Inquiry into the Genesis of Psychiatric Conditions in Early Childhood. *The Psychoanalytic Study of the Child* 1:53–74

TROP, J. (1988). Erotic and Eroticized Transference: A Self Psychology Perspective. *Psychoanalytic Psychology* 5:(3)269–284

TUCH. R. (2000). The Single Woman-Married Man Syndrome. Northvale, NJ: Jason Aronson.

——— (2007). Thinking With, and About, Patients Too Scared to Think. *Internatinoal Journal of Psychoanalysis* 88:91–111

WASKA, R. (1999). Oral Deprivation, Envy, and the Sadistic Aspects of the Ego. *Canadian Journal of Psychoanalysis* 7:(1)97–110

——— (2003). The Impossible Dream and the Endless Nightmare: Clinical Manifestations of Greed. *Canadian Journal of Psychoanalysis* 11:(2)379–397

WILSON. E. (1984). Love Among the Signifiers. *Psychoanalytic Inquiry* 4:(2)291–309.

END NOTES

1. Albert Mason, personal communication

2. Klein links the two phrases with the word "and," suggesting that the situation is always two-person in nature. This flies in the face of her other writings that clearly illustrate innate, internal issues at work. This leads me to believe that the word "and" is actually, in keeping with the rest of her writing, "and/or."

3. Imaging individuals to have selves that exist completely independent of context is a notion many have now gotten past.

4. This brings to mind the Peggy Lee song: "Is that all there is?"
5. This is the converse example of the projection of one's "nasty" traits—aggression, hostility, hate, etc.—that we had earlier entertained.

Richard Tuch
1800 Fairburn Avenue Ste. 206
Los Angeles, CA 90025
Rtuch@aol.com

Robert M. Galatzer-Levy

CHAPTER 5

Greed: Up Close and Personal

My theme in this paper is the psychology of the greedy individual. The impact of that greed on the social and economic surround will be, in a sense, a secondary matter. My point of view is from the inside of the individual rather than the effect it has on him from the external world. Psychoanalysts are made aware of how perspective shapes the perception of problems and situations daily. I look at greed from a perspective other than that usually taken by economists. Their discussions of greed start with the assumption that the wish to acquire wealth in arbitrarily large amounts is essentially rational. However, economists have become increasingly aware that actual behavior with regard to acquisition is often irrational because of the need to use heuristic rules of thumb, in making decisions.

The idea that it is always better to have more than less is not universally applicable. It is probably applicable only to those people who are aware of the possibilities that great wealth brings, such as the ability to establish large, long lasting institutions.

The Oxford English Dictionary says greed is "an *inordinate* or *insatiate longing*, especially for wealth-an avaricious or covetous *desire*. This definition does not focus on the acquisition of wealth *per se*. It focuses on the subjective state of an extreme, insatiable quality such that, no matter how much wealth an individual acquires, the need is never extinguished. It involves desire, a subjective feeling that it is urgent, like sensuous desire, not simply a rational dispassionate decision to acquire things.

Using this definition of greed, individual greed for money is clearly not always rational. Far from it. Repeated systematic studies indicate there is little or no evidence of a significant marginal increase in happiness or life satisfaction to having wealth beyond that which is needed to sustain a reasonable, whatever one defines as reasonable, lifestyle. People making \$10 million per annum are not by and large significantly either happier or more satisfied with their lives than people who are making \$80-thousand per annum.

Monetary greed is clearly different from the wish to acquire wealth, as indicated by the fact that getting too wealthy is often problematic.

People who greedily acquire objects soon discover that they do not have the space or time to enjoy them. Computations of the amount of money that people have to spend after they reach a certain level of wealth in order to keep the money reserves level and not accumulate more wealth, even if their money is very conservatively invested, indicate that one has to start spending at a rate that requires a great deal of effort. Indeed, to use relatively extreme examples, while it may sound lovely to have the house in Aspen, the house in Nantucket, the house in Newport Beach, and the house in the Bahamas, maintaining and organizing things to keep those four-to-ten houses operative is inordinately fatiguing. Wealth becomes in and of itself a burden regardless of how it is used.

As clinicians, we see that greedy people are quite often dominated by enormous fears of losing their wealth. They panic in situations where that wealth appears to be at risk. The well-documented irrationality of traders in the markets often demonstrates that they are profoundly panicked when it appears that their wealth may be disappearing. They become irrational in their efforts to maintain that wealth in essentially magical ways and lose the intellectual capacities for disciplined trading.

The emotional state of greed is commonly rationalized in terms of neoclassical economics. Rationalization is different from rationality. By rationalization, I mean disguising the emotional experience by a veneer of rationality. The fact that that veneer may be true does not alter the psychological reality of rationalization, that people are protecting themselves from the awareness of their internal psychological states.

It's easy to find dramatic examples of people whose greed has backfired. Ken Lay and Jeffrey Skilling were two men, as described in Bethany McLean's and Peter Elkind's book *The Smartest Guys in the Room: The Amazing Rise and Scandalous Fall of Enron* (2003), who dramatically illustrated how greed combined with grandiosity can have an enormous and horrific economic impact. As they are described both men suffered enormous stress and anxiety both on the way up and on the way down.

Economists in the past quarter century have approached the question of irrationality in a variety of ways because it is clear that the description of individuals acting purely rationally to acquire wealth does not explain a number of economic phenomenon. A few of these approaches should be mentioned.

Decision theorists such as Amos Tversky (2004) have demonstrated that in the situation of rapid change, in the situation where computation becomes difficult, we substitute so-called heuristic solutions, that is, rules of thumb, emotional impressions to make economic decisions. Naturally since these rules of thumb are, of necessity, just that, since the full computation that would be necessary cannot be made quickly enough and is not made, these solutions are less than rational. Precisely because the heuristic approach tends to be informal, often inarticulate and not thought through, they are liable to introduce systematic errors into economic thinking.

For example, as Dan Ariely (2008) has shown, the rule of thumb that it is very good to get something "free" operates powerfully. If given the offer to "buy one, get one free," people are so impressed by the opportunity to get something for nothing that they become entirely inattentive to the total cost of the transaction. Receiving a $4.00 box of cereal free when buying one at full price is regarded as much more attractive than receiving the same two boxes of cereal, each priced at $2.00.

A wonderful book by Harvard psychologist Daniel Gilbert called *Stumbling on Happiness* (2006) describes the pervasiveness of the use of heuristics in making decisions about the course of one's life and the inadequacy of these heuristics for this purpose. He discusses how people anticipate what will make them happy, and yet people are very bad at anticipating what they will find satisfying in the future. By and large, when we talk about what will make us happy in the future, we ask the question instead, "What would make us happy now?" and we start from that point, failing to realize that we are likely to be very different people at the point at which the decisions we make now will become operative.

Another direction that economists have taken is an appreciation of how individuals' consciously different motivations shape their economic actions, and we've heard some of this in terms of philanthropy. Speaking about conscious motives, George Akerlof, in his 2007 presidential address to the American Economic Association said of neoclassical economics theories that they have important motivations missing since they fail to incorporate the norms of the decision makers. These norms reflect how the respective decision makers think they and others should and should not behave. That is, Akerlof is arguing, that beyond acquisitiveness, moral values have a profound influence that shape the actual decisions that people make in the economic realm.

There is a long tradition of exploring economics in terms of noneconomic motives. Thorstein Veblen (1899), for example, argued that consumption is used as a way to gain and signal status. Marcel Mauss (1923) showed that exchange could be used primarily to increase social interaction and came to understand exchange largely in those terms. Karl Marx, especially in his 1844 manuscripts, discusses the experience of alienated labor, indicating how the lack of material engagement in production could be the cause of profound psychological distress.

In an earlier discussion of the ideas in this paper I was on a panel with Professor Robert Fogel, a Nobel Prize winning economist and historian who was, among other things, one of the founders of "cliometrics," the quantitative study of history. Fogel reviewed his ground-breaking work on the economics of American slavery, in which he had clearly demonstrated that African-American slaves were economically advantaged compared both to their African-American peers who had not been enslaved and to farming freemen in the American South. Much of this advantage resulted from the fact that, being property, these slaves were well treated to ensure that they maintained their value, for example, by not being physically injured so they could work. The tension that I think many of us felt as we listened to Professor Fogel's remarks was palpable. I thought, "This doesn't sound right. Why would we want to be a slaves?"

But why? According to Dr. Fogel's economic analysis, which I am sure is correct, slaves were better off in many contexts. So I titled the talk "Beyond Irrationality," because I think so far, the economic discussion of the factors that contribute to irrationality are not adequate, that greed is a more complicated matter than just an avowal of what one thinks one wants.

Freud and Klein explored greed as a derivative of early bodily concerns. With due respect to the psychoanalytic world, I think we have, so far, contributed relatively little to an understanding of the phenomenon of greed. Much of our language about bodily function with regard to the subject of greed and economics in general does not lead to the clarity of thinking that we want. It is incompletely explanatory, although it is very useful in being vivid. That is, the idea of the infant at the breast, the idea of hunger to such an extent that one feels as if one can never be satiated, nicely captures the emotional state of greedy individuals. So, too, the language of bodily experience, the terror of starvation, nicely put us in mind of the emotional state of the individual who is experiencing greed. But while these explanations get the affective intensity right, in actual analytic work they seldom seem to point to clear specific antecedents of adult greed.

There is an indirectly psychoanalytic contribution to economic thinking that has had a profound and practical influence. Edward Bernays,

Sigmund Freud's nephew, was the founder of modern public relations. He acknowledged his uncle's profound impact on his own thinking. Bernays clearly understood that economic decisions are made irrationally, that it is the task of public relations to understand empathically the state of mind of people and then to manipulate that state of mind.

I also come to the issue of perspective from the additional point of view derived from chaos and complexity theory. The connection between the activities of the individual and the emergent activities of the group is complex and difficult to predict. One of the major findings of complexity theory is that although autonomous agents may act according to some clear set of rules, those autonomous agents' actions are connected to what emerges when you bring a group of them together in a manner that is difficult to predict, or understand. It is hard to move either from the larger group phenomenon to the individual, or from the individual to the larger group.

Adam Smith's discovery of the function of markets is essentially the first discovery of how the activities of autonomous agents, each acting in a way that is not intended to accomplish a group phenomenon, can result in the emergence of economies and markets even though that is not their intention. Similarly, we know a great deal about how individual ants decide what to do, if decision is the right word. No individual ant decides to build an ant colony, yet these wonderful social insects develop these very complex structures.

I consider this important because even if we accept the idea that large-scale good often results from greed, this tells us very little about the state of mind of the individual greedy person. It does not tell us what it is like to be that ant who is carrying the bit of a leaf toward the ant hill, no matter how wonderful that ant hill may appear to be to an outside observer. Highly desirable outcomes for larger groups may result from highly undesirable outcomes for the individuals in the group. The idea that greed commonly results in greater productivity is from a macroeconomic point of view a good thing. This idea is perfectly consistent with the idea that the individuals involved in enacting greed are chronically distressed.

So let us turn to the psychological question of greed as this inordinate, insatiable need for more in an economic arena. The word greed itself comes from the shortening of the Old English (*grǣdig*). Greedy is simply a word denoting hunger.

I hope you will forgive me for not presenting clinical data at this point. Every analyst, I think, has considerable opportunity to observe greed up close and personal. Unfortunately, the best examples of these phenomena are not such that one can present them publicly without seriously violating the confidentiality of the individuals involved. So I'm going to use some examples from literature to examine greed, and I will ask you to be patient with my failure to provide genuine and clinically close empirical data, which I will tell you exists, but which I will not use today.

I will instead use Charles Dickens' Scrooge to illustrate my point. I would ordinarily be reluctant to choose a literary exemplar of the phenomenon that is so one-dimensional a character because real people ordinarily have a complexity that is missed in such overly simple representation. Yet Scrooge is universally recognized. Every reader knows Scrooge, has an image of him, and feels him to have a significant psychological reality. This suggests that Dickens captured something in his depiction of him. In this instance the character's one-dimensional quality is not the result of Dickens' failure to develop the character fully but rather it is a central quality of the character himself. Scrooge's greed overwhelms all other aspects of his character. Those of us who have worked with the Scrooges of the world know that the inordinate preoccupation with wealth commonly overshadows every other aspect of their lives. Relations with other people, aesthetic and sensuous pleasures, conscious fantasies and dreams are pervaded with money, its accumulation and its display.

Let us look at some of Scrooge's qualities. Clearly Scrooge is unhappy. His acquisition of money gives him little or no pleasure even though he values it over everything else. His greed is intimately connected to his misanthropy and his envious hatred of those who have intimate personal relations. What Scrooge is missing is a relationship with other human beings and he finds no way to have it. So he envies and detests those who do.

We learn from Dickens that Scrooge's miserliness originates in the loss of his relationship with his fiancée. He has lost a relationship which provided something of great necessity, and he is now chronically engaged in trying to make up for that loss through the acquisition of wealth. He has also lost his business partner, Morley—who was rather like Scrooge in some ways—and he is alone in the world when we encounter him at the beginning of *A Christmas Carol*.

If we look at the histories of individuals who exhibit the kind of greed that I am talking about, we often see some kind of loss. The obvious kind of loss of a parent or a loved one is common enough, but even more common is the loss of the experience of an early caretaking environment. Ken Lay, for example, grew up in not just an economically bleak environment, but also in a profoundly emotionally bleak world, an environment devoid of tenderness and care Clinically one finds these to be a common denominator of the greedy.

Now let's look at another literary character, Scrooge's namesake, Walt Disney's cartoon, *Uncle Scrooge McDuck* (for illustrations and more information, see www.en.wikipedia.org/wiki/Scrooge_McDuck).

The first comic in which Scrooge McDuck appears was published in 1947. He says of himself, obviously angry, his teeth gnashed, "Me, I'm different. Everybody hates me, and I hate everybody" (Barks 1947). Walt Disney, who may have known about these matters internally, recognized the intimate relationship between greed and a hatred and anger toward the world and other people. Scrooge McDuck also engages in something close to a perversion with money. That is, he derives sensuous pleasure from it: He is repeatedly portrayed having lustful, sensuous experience with his money—diving into his money, running money through his fingers. It is like watching a kind of pornography that you cannot quite get into, the kinds of pornography one looks at and wonders, "Why would anyone want to do that?" This response not only reflects reaction formation, perhaps to the obvious anality of Scourge's lust, but that the sexuality is preserve in the sense that its aim is not bodily or aesthetic pleasure and its object is not human.

Another depiction of Uncle Scrooge points to an important aspect of greed. It is often accompanied by anxiety. One expression of Scrooge McDuck, which is fairly typical of him, indicates a kind of distress and worry coincident with his monetary delight.

Now how are we to understand these phenomena? Psychoanalyst Heinz Kohut (1968) addressed the question, "What happens when, for whatever reason, the personality in some way disintegrates, or when there is a threat of disintegration, or when the sense of vitality is lost or threatened?" He recognized that such states are probably the most distressing states that most people will experience. He also recognized that the cohesiveness of the self is ordinarily supported through relationships with other people.

Each of the greedy characters I have discussed so far has impoverished interpersonal relationships. Their interpersonal relations do not work well enough to keep them feeling coherent and whole. In the face of potential fragmentation, we often see a frantic attempt to reconstitute the self or reconstitute some sense of coherence and meaning. This is aimed at constructing some substitution for the interpersonal relations that might have otherwise supported the individual's sense of being alive and whole. Kohut referred to such attempts as "fragmentation products."

Greed may be usefully conceptualized as a fragmentation product, that is, an attempt to reconstitute the fragmented self, or to maintain a sense of self in the face of the potential loss of coherence. It is an attempt at a solution of the problem of, "How do you feel alive? How do you feel coherent in the face of the lack of opportunity to feel coherence in the more ordinary way of having the interactions and supports with other human beings?"

The desperate search is for a sense of organization, coherence, and comfort. If we look at the phenomenology of greed, we see many indications that there is a loss of coherence. There is a disappearance, or relative disappearance of an interest in other people, as manifest in the ruthlessness of many greedy individuals. It suggests that while in the thrall of greed, their experience of others is such that the idea that other people even exist—and are to be considered as human beings—has been lost. This loss of the experience of other persons as human and the appropriate objects of empathy helps explain why greed is so often accompanied by moral turpitude. If the foundation of moral behavior toward other people rests in the recognition that they are feeling beings like oneself, the loss of the experience of others as fully human makes it easier to be indifferent to them and to treat them badly.

There is often a loss of an integrated sense of moral concern, which easily leads to corruption. The ease with which panic and distress emerge—for example, the impairment of a capacity to sooth oneself that is commonly seen in greedy individuals and the panic associated with economic setbacks—is more evidence that the self is no longer functioning as a coherent effective whole. The loss of sound judgment that we commonly see in people who are greedy, the years and years of systematic effort going down the drain as a person says, "I have to win this one. I have to not lose this time," is an indication of how little the connection to reality can be in the face of the fragmentation that I am suggesting underlines much of greed.

Finally, the isolation and compartmentalization of experience, sometimes called splitting, such that greedy individuals can, at times, be kind, and interested can exist in parallel with, and not be affected by, the sense that, "I must get money regardless of the consequences for others." This kind of vertical splitting, that Kohut described, is seen very commonly in greedy people.

Greed arises from the urgent sense of needing something that will provide the functions of the coherent self. It arises within a context of a sense of hopelessness about getting what one really needs in human ways.

The phenomena associated with greed were actually studied very long before Kohut. They are described quite wonderfully, if in somewhat strange language by Melanie Klein (1957), a Hungarian woman who founded a major school of psychoanalysis in Britain. Her analysand and student, Wilfred Bion, extended and elaborated her ideas to the study of thinking in a manner that will be particularly useful in thinking about greed. Klein and Bion both emphasized how fragmented mental states involve failures in thinking or breakdowns in thinking.

There is a particularly interesting way in which this occurs. Ordinarily we think in symbols. That is, we observe the world and then engage in mental operations on representations of the world. These representations under appropriate operations maintain significant aspects of the situation in the external world. For example, if I think about my relationship to my children, I have a mental picture of my children. If I am fortunate, it is a relatively rich picture of them. This relatively complex picture of them includes the multiple and various ways in which I feel and respond to them, the multiple and various ways in which they feel and respond to me, and the context of history that we have had. I can use these representations to think about them and my relationship to them—anticipating the consequences of various actions on my part in order to plan for successful interactions or avoid unfortunate ones, evoking them in situations where they are physically absent to provide pleasure or solace, etc.

But in states of distress, Klein and Bion argue, there is a breakdown in this process of symbol formation so that instead of having rich symbols, we are simply left with signs or tokens of what once were images of people. These symbols are subject to further and problematic degradation. For example, overly simplified or distorted pictures of individuals may emerge.

Tokens to be used as money were first developed in ancient Mesopotamia. Now for economic purposes, the development of tokens was a major step forward. That is, if I want to exchange twelve sheep for twenty units of wheat, if I have to haul around all those sheep and all that wheat to make the exchange, the process will be inordinately complicated. On the other hand, if I can exchange tokens to achieve the same end the process is quite simple.

So the invention of tokens, the beginnings of money, made economic exchange far easier. However, there is a little difficulty that comes in at this point. That is, psychologically, although the token is only valuable insofar as it represents the sheep or the wheat, I can begin to make a split, a division in my thinking, in which the token becomes of value in and of itself. There is an opportunity for a kind of confusion that results, an opportunity that makes possible a kind of breakdown in which out of anxiety or out of stupidity I forget that this thing is not a sheep. It is a piece of clay and it has no intrinsic value. It is only valuable insofar as it can be exchanged for a sheep. But this knowledge can easily become elusive.

In greed, one of the phenomenon that occurs as part of the overall breakdown I am describing is that there is a replacement of symbols with signs. There is a replacement of things, which stand for other things and are known clearly to stand for other things with a fascination with the object that should stand for something else. The money itself becomes valuable. We hear this, for example, in common figures of speech.

When we say someone is worth $5 million, what do we mean? Well, literally what we mean is that their wealth is $5 million. But that is not the way it is actually used. The person's value is in some sense is measured in these quantities which are wholly inappropriate for measuring human worth. There has been a disconnection between the token and the thing it stands for.

The phenomenon mentioned earlier of acquiring wealth to the extent that one is burdened by that wealth and has to spend all one's time somehow managing to spend it, that problem can only occur when there's a disconnect between the idea of money and what one can do with money.

The core of greed involves a first a step in which the self is threatened with fragmentation, followed by a shift in cognition in which what should be symbols are deprived of their meaning, and having lost their meaning, become valued in themselves. There is only one trouble. No matter how many sheep tokens I have, I cannot get one ounce of wool from them unless I use them in their symbolic form as a medium of exchange. I can have 20,000 tokens of sheep and I cannot get a lamb chop out of it unless I am able to transform it.

So if I said to myself, "I will gather to myself as many sheep as I am able," I can never be satisfied if I gather these tokens. I can never have the experiences associated with having actual sheep. We see this, I think, clinically in individuals who must gather more and more in the hope of getting what they need, but repeatedly discover that it cannot possibly satisfy them, hence, the hunger remains. It is like eating food that has no nutritional value. You remain hungry forever.

What is one to do in the face of greed if we understand greed as a breakdown product that goes through this special mechanism of the loss of meaning of symbols for exchange? We have, again, a wonderful literary example in George Eliot's *Silas Marner* (1861). Those of you who read *Silas Marner* in middle school should pick it up again as adults, because it is a far, far better book than you may remember it as being.

The history of Silas Marner begins with a breakdown. That is, Marner is in a situation where he loses not only his beloved—in this instance, another man—but also he loses the community of which he is a part. For that, he substitutes the idea of collecting wealth of various kinds, particularly gold, and he desperately needs this gold.

Now through the vicissitudes that can only occur in novels, his gold is lost. He is confronted, however, with an infant who has some similarity to the gold, that is her golden hair reminds Marner of the material gold which he has lost. The book is largely dedicated to the rediscovery by Marner of human relations, the rediscovery that he can have a sense of happiness in the Aristotelian sense of satisfaction by virtue of having a relationship to another human being, particularly poignantly by virtue of having the relationship in which he facilitates another person's development into maturity.

What occurs by virtue of this is that he is cured of his greed. He's no longer greedy, because he has found a route to genuine satisfaction in personal relations.

Most of us, and most greedy people, do not have lives which conform to the plotline of a novel written by a compassionate author, and so most of us have limited opportunities in life to have the kind of developmental discovery that Silas Marner has. The psychoanalysis of individuals who are greedy often has the same transformative effect. It promotes the discovery or rediscovery of the centrality of relations to other people providing what it is one is really hungry for, what it is one really desires, and the recognition that the substitute satisfactions of money inevitably cannot work.

This is the core of the analytic work with many greedy individuals. Commonly people with histories of greed, or experiences of greed, will come to analysis precisely for the reason that they discover it is not working, the acquisition of yet more wealth leaves them with a sense of emptiness and triviality, disorganization, incoherence, which is nearly intolerable. So the analytic setup can be used to provide a new experience of a relationship, which provides actual meaning to their lives instead of the greedy acquisition of things, which can never truly satisfy.

I want to emphasize that this discussion of greed, comes out of a perspective of looking at the psychology of the greedy individual. It does not negate other perspectives but it certainly suggests that greed cannot be described as a unitary matter, that the problematic aspect of greed is not simply that it has a negative effect on other people, but that greed reflects an internal state of great psychological but treatable distress.

REFERENCES

ARIELY, D. (2008). *Predictably Irrational: The Hidden Forces That Shape Our Decisions.* New York: HarperCollins.

AKERLOF, G. (2007). The Missing Motivation in Macroeconomics www.aeaweb.org/annual_mtg_papers/2007/0106_1640_0101.pdf.

BARKS, C. (1947). Christmas on Bear Mountain. in *Four Color Comics,* #178, New York: Dell Comics.

ELIOT, G. (1861). *Silas Marner.* Edinburgh & London: William Blackwood and Sons.

GILBERT, D. (2006*). Stumbling on Happiness.* New York: A.A. Knopf.

MCLEAN, B. & ELKIN, P. (2003). *The Smartest Guys in the Room: The Amazing Rise and Scandalous Fall of Enron.* New York: Portfolio Hardcover.

KOHUT, H. (1968). The Psychoanalytic Treatment of Narcissistic Personality Disorders: Outline of a Systematic Approach. *Psychoanalytic Study of the Child* 23:86–113.

KLEIN, M. (1957). *Envy and Gratitude A Study of Unconsious Sources.* New York: Basic Books.

MARX, K., (1844) *The Economic and Philosophic Manuscripts of 1844 and the Communist Manifesto* Transl. M. Mulligan, Amherst, NY:Prometheus Books, 1988.

MAUSS, M. (1923). *The Gift: The Form and Reason for Exchange in Archaic Societies.* Transl, W.D. Halls, New York: W.W. Norton, 2000.

TVERSKY, A. (2004). *Preference, Belief, and Similarity: Selected Writings,* ed. Eldar Shafir. Cambridge, MA: The MIT Press.

VEBLEN, T. (1899). *The Theory of the Leisure Class.* New York: Penguin, 1994.

Robert M. Galatzer-Levy
Gala@uchicago.edu

Arlene Kramer Richards

CHAPTER 6

GAMBLING AND DEATH

Those—dying then
Knew where they went—
They went to God's Right Hand—
That Hand is amputated now
And God cannot be found—

The abdication of Belief—
Makes the Behavior small—
Better an ignis fatuus
Than no illume at all

—EMILY DICKINSON, 1882

Emily Dickinson trembles at the idea of a world with no supreme being because there is no alternative to death in such a world. There is no guarantee of justice. Chaos is unbearable. She asks for a false god rather than no first principle at all. This paper is about the false god of gambling—a God that some find irresistible when confronted with the death of those they love. There are no odds to death. Everyone dies.

The comforting thing about gambling games is that there are rules, the gambler knows the odds ahead of time—and there are odds. Like death, losing at a casino is inevitable, but on the way to that loss, everything is fair.

In an earlier paper (Richards & Richards 1997) written with Arnold Richards, we showed how Las Vegas, the mecca of the gambling world in mid twentieth century, was a vast temple dedicated to denying death. Three movies about Las Vegas showed how the gambler denies his own death. *Bugsy* (1991) showed how Bugsy Siegel created Las Vegas and died for breaking the rules; the movie *Casino* (1995) showed how a character named "Ace Rosenthal" industrialized Las Vegas and died for breaking the rules; and a movie called *Leaving Las Vegas* (1995) showed a loser who accepts the lack of odds and comes to Las Vegas in order to die. Like those who come to Las Vegas to gamble now, the characters in these movies accept their inevitable deaths, but at the same time live as if they know the rules and by keeping to them, they can prevent their own deaths. In this paper I want to extend that theme to show how gambling enables denial of the death of those the gambler loves.

The Movies

In the movie *21* (2008), a group of MIT students is recruited to count cards at Las Vegas for the game of 21. A touching moment of connection shows the young hero with the girl of his dreams who is already a member of the group to which he is being recruited. She tells him about how her father taught her the game, and when he asks about her father, she tells him that he is long gone. His father has been dead for many years as well. Not only does this make it clear that they are going to be lovers, it also makes it clear that the students were fascinated by gambling for a reason. Death ties them to each other and death makes gambling fascinating. What makes the hero love his experience in Vegas is not explained in any other way—this is enough.

It is interesting to compare this with the book on which the movie is based. Called *Bringing Down the House* (Mezrich 2001), the book is a non-fiction "as-told-to" tale of gambling and yet not gambling, only seeming to gamble. And a striking difference between the movie and the book is that the hero of the book has a living father. His father is a successful scientist, as he wants his son to be. But the book describes the son as lonely in his lab, cut off from the living world. Invited to join a glamorous group of fellow students by a charismatic professor, he gladly gives up his scientific career for the gambling life. By counting the cards that have already been played in the deck they can figure out when high cards are likely to come up and then bet accordingly. The point is that they use statistics—a science that was actually invented for gambling—to ensure that they will have the advantage over the house; they will win eventually. The purpose of devoting their considerable talents to this, rather than to science or mathematics is the thrill of being in the moment, not in preparing for a long distant future, not in thinking of the past experience with family, friends, teachers, classmates, but being in the moment with a group of people also there only for the moment.

Yet the book and the movie both center around scenes of the pseudo-gamblers actually gambling with their lives as they defy the house rules against counting cards in the casino. They know that the casino owners can be dangerous. They have heard stories of card counters being mugged and of others disappearing into the desert. An older gambler warns them:

"Don't let some guy named Vinnie take you on any long drives out into the desert" (p. 73).

They are not gambling at the 21 game, they are gambling with their lives. The knowledge that they are not gamblers in the card game is offset by the thrill of being on the edge, facing what may be the last moment of their lives.

In one interview in both book and movie a woman gambler says: "I found the thrill of the game almost as addictive as the field of consulting. The idea of going up against a huge corporation, finding ways to beat them in their own arena—it was a real high." (p. 124). The interviewer says: "I nodded. I had heard this from everyone on the team. They all saw themselves as little Davids going up against a giant, neon Goliath. Except in their version, David got rich off the battle" (p. 125).

For the woman interviewed, as for the other gamblers, the money was only a token. And the games are played with tokens, reinforcing the difference between the money in gambling and the money used to pay for tangible goods. For real gamblers the token is exchanged for money. For these counters the token stands for life. The interviewer does not see that in the bible story David not only gets rich, he also gets to keep his life and he gets to be king. In other words, what makes the thrill is the heroic stand against the more powerful force. David risked his life. Gambling is a thrill when life is the stake. Another thrill was dressing up for the casino experience. The MIT students went to Las Vegas dressing up as ordinary gamblers, impersonating people from whom the casino could expect to make money. The game of being different from themselves added to the fun. They were like children dressing up for Halloween with the fun and death-defying bravado of pretending. The movie makes it clear that the actual gamblers the MIT team was impersonating also chose special outfits, make-up, hairstyles to create personas for the purpose of impressing the other people at the casino. These impersonations are more glamourous than real life and reinforce the pretence of the casino, the idea that one has not suffered and will not suffer loss. Jeff Ma is the central character in the book. At the end of the second edition of the book the author interviews him about his family and friends' reactions to the story. Jeff says:

"But now, well, the reaction has all been pretty positive. I think people understand that the ethics of what we were doing—well, it wasn't like we were going to Vegas to gamble. We were using math to beat the system" (p. 260).

He is now out of danger and again in denial of he real risk he took. His loss of the woman he loved is never mentioned—though he clearly understands that his gambling destroyed their intimacy. In the after interview he mentions what the gambling got him: a townhouse and a share in a bar. He does not mention having a new relationship. For him, as for other gamblers, the group around the table is the level of intimacy they want. Winning or losing is almost beside the point, being in the situation is what they prize above intimacy. Once the person that the gambler loved is lost, gambling replaces her and replaces any regrets he might have had about losing her.

A Book

But the idea of a system to beat the odds is a very common one among gamblers. It is the point of a gambling addiction. The gambler must believe that he or she can beat the system. In Dostoyevsky's *The Gambler* (1866), two very different gamblers use two very different systems. Both lose. A third person at the gambling tables is "the old lady." But the old lady gambles by betting with the house. She accepts her inability to escape death by gambling. Early in the novel death is introduced when the narrator, the gambler, asks the woman he loves what has happened since he last saw her:

"Nothing, but the arrival of two pieces of news from St. Petersburg, first, that Granny was very ill, and then, two days later, that she seemed to be dying" (p. 11).

This statement outlines the plot of the entire novel. A group of gamblers, their dependents and those to whom they are in debt, are waiting for the death and for the money that they will inherit, swindle or be repaid. Tragic and comedic at the same time, the novel focusses on the addiction to gambling as a way of denying time, death, and the loss for which the odds are inescapable. The gambler who is the hero and narrator of the novel, makes a first attempt at explaining it sociologically:

> The Russian is not only incapable of amassing capital, but dissipates it in a reckless and unseemly way. Nevertheless we Russians need money, too, . . . and consequently we are very glad to make use of such means as roulette, for instance, in which one can grow rich all at once, in two hours, without work That's very fascinating to us; and since we play badly, recklessly, without taking trouble, we usually lose. (p. 32).

Life with its tiny increments of time—and work with its tiny increments of achievement, earning, and saving with very slow gains—are of no interest to a gambler. What he values is the moment in which time seems suspended, the moment between placing the bet and finding the outcome. Death is what comes in a moment; life is a tedious step-by-step journey. In the novel the Granny, rather than dying and leaving her money to the gamblers, becomes a gambler herself and loses her money. The gamblers had counted on her death as a way to get money with which to continue gambling. The death of a supportive and protective family member is shown as a necessary condition for gambling.

The gambler in the title of the book goes down the gambling road to the end. Dostoyevsky's *The Gambler* describes the experience of the moment from the inside. While writing this novel, Dostoyevsky was also writing *Crime and Punishment* (1866). He was deeply in debt, had been to debtor's prison already and was facing it again. He had contracted to deliver two novels by a certain date. If he did not deliver on time, the publisher would own all of Dostoyevsky's future writings. He would never be able to make his living by writing again. Gambling that he could finish the novel by the given date, he was rushing to finish it in what was in effect a life-or-death struggle. In the novel, the old lady of the gambling table chooses to return to ordinary life in which she will, as Dostoyevsky himself finally did, seek immortality through religion rather than at the card table. As he describes it in Crime and Punishment, the choice of religion is a choice of connection with others, a salvation through love. It is the opposite of the choice Jeff Ma makes in *21.*

Gambling in a casino is a spectator sport. The players watch each other, on any one play they are surrounded by watchers. Dressing in particularly eye catching costumes, make-up, hairdos and jewelry is part of the play. Dostoyevsky shows it this way:

> "I watched you ma'am," Marfa cackled, and said to Potapitch, "What does our lady want to do?" And the money on the table—saints alive! the money! I haven't seen so much money in the whole of my life, and all around were gentlefolk—nothing but gentlefolk sitting. "And wherever do all these gentlefolk come from Potapitch?" said I. "May Our Lady herself help her," I thought. "I was praying for you ma'am," and my heart was simply sinking, simply sinking, I was all of atremble. "Lord help her," I thought, "and here the Lord has sent you luck, I've been trembling ever since, ma'am, I'm all of a tremble now" (p. 101).

Like the spectators in Las Vegas, those in Dostoyevsky's Roulette-ville admire the elegance of the players, feel trembling and hope as if they were lovers anticipating orgasm, and trembling afterward as if they had been moved to orgasm and were now coming down to everyday reality from it. If orgasm is the "little death," gambling is the public orgasm, the public little death.

The gambler himself experiences losing all his money as if it were a death: "What am I now? Zero. What may I be tomorrow? Tomorrow I may rise from the dead and begin to live again!" (p. 170). The zero is particularly apt as it is the number in roulette in which everyone's money goes to the bank. All players lose except those who have bet on zero. Plainly only the bank can win. In the end, the bank always wins. Death is inevitable. But the moment before death is worth dying for. The moment when it is still possible that the gambler and not the bank will win this time. And that moment is to the gambler better than the moment of orgasm, the moment that also just precedes death.

Once having experienced the death and rebirth at the gambling table, the gambler no longer wants sexual fulfillment as much as he wants the gambling high moment. In the novel, a Mr. Astley comes to the gambler a year after that first moment and offers him the love of the woman for whom he was gambling in the first place. Astley is the symbol of British prudence. He confronts the gambler :

> You have not only given up life, all your interests, private and public, the duties of a man and a citizen, your friends (and you really had friends)—you have not only given up your objects, such as they were, all but gambling—you have even given up all your memories.

The gambler answers:

> "Enough, Mr, Astley, please, don't remind me," I cried with vexation, almost with anger, "let me tell you, I've forgotten absolutely nothing; but I've only for a time put everything out of my mind, even my memories, until I can make a radical improvement in my circumstances, then . . . .then you will see, I shall rise again from the dead" (p. 174).

What he will do when he rises from the dead is to go back to his beloved. He will return to human intimacy. To be resurrected, to be returned from the dead is the promise of religion, in these accounts, the false religion of gambling promises the gambler a new life in which he wins the love of the beautiful woman rather than the death of losing everything to the House.

A Memoir

Double Down is a memoir (Bartheme & Barthelme 1999) linking gambling and death. Its authors are brothers, both successful academics and writers. In their book they describe how they managed to lose a quarter of a million dollars, all the money they had inherited from their ambivalently loved father. They observe: "Our fellow gamblers were serious, not like academics but in the furious way that children are serious, concentrating on play, oblivious, intense, yet at ease Essentially, they came to the casino to be children" (p. 74).

The authors, like their fellow gamblers, were acting like they were still children, living in the time before their father died. As they describe it their fantasy was: "Things would suddenly and inexplicably turn in our favor. A hurricane of money and love" (p .85). Gambling enabled them to escape the reality of their father's death:

> Gambling is of course, a very expensive way to beat reason. You can get pretty much the same thing by staying awake for a night and a day, or however long it takes you to get a little psychologically unhinged, destabilized, detached from whatever you believed the day before, and then staring at the cat, the dog, the stapler, the back of your hand, water. Most anything will do once you've shed your silly confidence. (p. 97).

Knowing that gambling at a casino was rigged so that over time they had to lose, they tried to understand what they were doing:

> . . . we were more serious, more ardent in our courtship of loss. We practiced, we tried harder, we dumped the cash our father had tried so hard to put together for us. Was the message clear? Was it, "We don't want your money"? Or was it, "Consider yourself repudiated"? Or was it more like, "Thanks for this chance to feel like a loser on a large scale"? Or was it, "This money is a poor substitute for you"? (pp. 116–117)

I think that the answer is one that multiple choice tests provide: All of the above. But the gamble is not only about losing. Winning provides much of the same feeling:

> The losing part is not fun exactly, in fact, fun doesn't come into it. but the heat, the dizzying adrenal rush, is much the same whether the chips come back to you, or go into the dealer's rack. . . . play the game, any game, for significant stakes and you'll know. It's not whether you win or lose, its that you play. (pp. 118–119).

The brothers come to understand that: "We lost the money because we played, because we wouldn't give up, because giving up was unheard of, because our parents were dead and there was no order to our lives" (p. 136).

They talk as if gambling would put order in their lives, as if the rules of the game are the important thing, the "ignus fatuus" of Dickinson's poem, the false god that comforts even when the believer knows that the god is false. The brothers only stop gambling when they are kicked out of the casino Like the players in 21, the rules of harsh reality supersede those of the magical gambling world, the veil is torn away, the wizard turns out to be a poor reminder that death does exist, human life is finite and the odds do not apply. There is no escape. Everybody loses the people they love.

A psychoanalytic understanding of death has been late in coming. The idea of a death instinct as posited first by Spielrein (1912) and elaborated by Freud (1920), has been rejected by the ego psychologists. The idea of death as one of the feared calamities of childhood was controversial when posited as annihilation anxiety by Hurvich (1989). The idea that a person defends against the threat of death by manic defense fits with the psychology of gambling as I have outlined it here. In the end, gambling provides moments of immediacy of sensation that shut out fears of all kinds, fears of being abandoned, of being excluded, of losing one's powers, and of being deprived of the exclusive love of one's parents. But each of these fears is made concrete in the thought of parental death. These depictions of gambling in fiction, non-fiction and semi-fictional film show the ways gambling fends off the thoughts, feelings and images evoked by the possibility of death.

Freud described a gambling game in "The Theme of Three Caskets." Here the caskets are used as if they were shells in a shell game. He who chooses the golden casket loses, He who chooses the silver casket also loses, and the one who chooses the lead casket wins. Freud understands the gold to represent the woman who gives birth to the man, the silver casket to represent the wife who loves him and the lead casket as representing the Lady Death. Of these varieties of love, the ultimate winner is Death.

If death is the ultimate lover is the death of a loved one a betrayal? Does the survivor wonder: "Did the one I love love death more than he or she loved me?" In the first hand account of the death of her husband and the year she spent mourning him, Didion (2005) attempts to:

> . . . make sense of the period that followed [the death], weeks and then months that cut loose any fixed idea I ever had about death, about illness, about probability and luck, about good fortune and bad, about marriage and children and memory, about grief, about the ways people do and do not deal with the fact that life ends, about the shallowness of sanity, about life itself (p. 7).

A remarkable feature of the book is her constant reference to the dates of events, important events like weddings and adoption, public events like assassination of a president, all attached to numbers, all ordered mathematically. The whole book is like a statistical manual, a gambler's memoir, a record of luck, both good and bad. It makes clear how the obsessional defense fits into the gambling activity and the card counting "not gambling" activity of the professional MIT players as a strategy to defeat the death of a loved person.

REFERENCES

BARTHELME, F. & BARTHELME, S. (1999). *Double Down.* New York: Harcourt.

CAROTENUTO, A.(1982; 1983). *A Secret Symmetry: Sabina Spielrein between Jung and Freud.* New York: Pantheon Books

DIDION, J. (2005). *The Year of Magical Thinking.* New York: Knopf.

DOSTOYEVSKY, F. (1866). The Gambler. Transl. C. Garnett, ed G.S. Morson. New York: Modern Library, 2003.

——— (1866). *Crime and Punishment.* Transl. D. McDuff, New York: Penguin, 2002.

FREUD, S. (1912). The Theme of The Three Caskets. *Standard Edition* 12:289–301.

——— (1920). Beyond the pleasure principle. *Standard Edition* 18:7–43.

HAYMAN, R. (2001). *A Life of Jung.* New York: W W Norton & Company.

HURVICH,. M. (1989). Traumatic Moment, Basic Dangers, and Annihilation Anxiety. *Psychoanalytic Psychology.* 6:309–323.

MEZRICH, B. (2002) *21: Bringing Down the House: The Inside Story of Six MIT Students Who Took Vegas for Millions*. New York: Free Press.

RICHARDS, A.K., & RICHARDS, A.D. (1997). Gambling, Death and Violence: Hollywood Looks at Las Vegas. *Psychoanalytic Review* 84:769–788.

SPIELREIN, S. (1912). Die Destruktion Als Ursache Des Werdens. *Jahrbuch der Psychoanalyse* 4; English Transl. Destruction as a Cause of Becoming. by S.K. Witt (1995) in *Psychoanalysis and Contemporary Thought* 18:85–118.

Arlene Kramer Richards
200 East 89th Street
New York, NY 10128
arlenerichards89@gmail.com

Leslie Shaw CHAPTER 7

A Psychodynamic Perspective on The Financial Crisis

During the recent months as financial events have unfolded some of you in the audience may have been reminded, as I have been, of the famous Claude Rains remark in the movie *Casablanca* (1942). We are shocked to see what is happening here; to realize what appears to have become so ubiquitous around us?

But I believe that one of the aspirations that we (psychoanalysts) should have, especially in the midst of these events, is to try to size psychoanalytic thinking and ideas for a more broad audience than we have typically been able to reach in the past. And so with that approach in mind, from a psychoanalytic point-of-view, we might pause to ask: Is there an inner logic to this crisis phenomenon that has occurred? Certainly there is a repetition that keeps going on the corrupt events about which we have become so aware, never mind the ones that have not yet been revealed but are sure to come.

Among the things that I hope to communicate to you today is that academic economics, for all of its rigor in the past 250 years, has excluded any recognition of unconscious meaning as having any explanatory contribution or purpose to economic or financial decision making. And we should think especially of this even with the academic superstars who have become the President's economic team. Moreover the genuine success, since the 1970s, of the cognitive and behavioral psychologies contributions to economic decisions still leaves us wanting of any unifying model between economic endeavors and the breadth or depth of our humanity. The behavioral psychology discipline that has allied with economics in the past three decades explains man's mental limitations in terms of something called "bounded rationality". The behavioral focus is on humans' inability to process complex information as a basis for peoples' failure to anticipate disasters such as this current one. And to a considerable extent the idea of bounded rationality is a correct one.

But I prefer today to emphasize a *paradox* between all of our exposed economic dysfunctions, corruptions and their link to our humanity.

And I want to suggest that we can enhance the human contribution to the "bounded" part of rationality. In order to get to this paradoxical view I need to set-the-stage for you with a couple of historical stories about the development of economic theory.

The first is about the economist Adam Smith who published the most influential economics book of all time, in the mid-1760s: It was titled *An Inquiry into the Nature and Causes of the Wealth of Nations* (1776). Its influence on the studies of economics and on our daily lives is as if it had been passed into law. Ask anyone what the book is about and likely the answer will be that it is about "competition". It marked the discovery of the "invisible hand" which is the supposed self-organizing system of prices and quantities that we know today as the price system. But there was also a second insight in the *Wealth of Nations* having to do with scale and specialization. The second insight, often called the "pin factory," showed that if employees specialized on narrow defined tasks, they could produce far more than they could if each worked independently. What is not obvious at first is the way that these two concepts stand in opposition to each other. The parable of the pin factory says that there are increasing returns to scale, the bigger the factory. Yet increasing returns create a tendency toward monopoly; that is to say, a tendency to acquire more specializations.

And for the earlier insight, the invisible hand, to work properly there must be many competitors in each industry so that nobody is in a position to exert monopoly power. Therefore, the ideas that free markets always get it right depends on the assumption that returns to scale are diminishing, not increasing.

For almost two centuries, economic thinking was dominated by the assumption of diminishing returns, with the Pin Factory pushed into the background. Why? It wasn't about ideology but rather it was about following the line of least mathematical *resistance*. Diminishing returns lend themselves readily to elegant mathematical formalism but increasing returns are notoriously hard to represent in the form of a mathematical model. Yet over the decades (and centuries) increasing returns were always a conspicuous part of reality. There was a consistent repetition of their appearance in the scheme of things. Nevertheless, they did not get brought in to the mainstream of economic thought. In commenting on this history some years ago, the Nobel Laureate Kenneth Arrow (Arrow, Yew-Kwang, & Xiaokai 1998) was the first to remark openly that increasing returns were always "an underground river" in economic thought. They were always there. Yet they rarely saw the light of day. Throughout economic history the problem would "bubble-up" to the surface, only to be discarded again for lack of a rigorous, clear or certain way to include them. *So within the history of rational economics we seem to have a symptomatic repetition compulsion.*

Now, before I leave this vignette about the history of economic theory and Adam Smith I want to emphasize that Smith had written a book, eight years prior to the *Wealth of Nations*. The earlier work was titled: *The Theory of Moral Sentiments* (1759). Its essence, briefly, can be captured directly from it: "How selfish so ever man may be supposed, there are certainly some principles in his nature which interest him in the fortunes of others, and render their happiness necessary to him, though he derives nothing except the pleasure of seeing it". Later he adds: "the chief part of human happiness arises from the consciousness of being beloved". Other aspects of the book beautifully discuss human emotional frailty and Adam Smith's fear that "reason, when wedded to human frailty, can lead to destructive interpersonal conflict," for if it is unbridled, self-interest drives each of us to seek a larger share of the human bounty for ourselves.

Respected scholars of Adam Smith record that Smith tried to work the Moral Sentiments into the *Wealth of Nations*. He devoted a section of "Wealth" to an extended synthesis of the original Moral Sentiments work. Nevertheless after the *Wealth of Nations* appeared, with its unnoticed contradiction between diminishing and increasing returns, the book that was Smith's *Theory of Moral Sentiments* eventually became all but forgotten.

The second historical story to share with regard to the paradox of economic dysfunction and its link to our humanity is more brief yet important.

All of the *repression* of the so-called underground river of increasing returns that kept bubbling up in economic reality was a repetition phenomena that continued throughout the nineteenth and well into the twentieth centuries. Yet during these centuries there was considerable collaboration on other fronts taking place between economists and psychologists, especially in the nineteenth century. Throughout those years discounting of the future was explained psychologically in terms of motivational effects. This evolved later to cognition being a definer in the relation between psychology and economics. The basic idea was trade-offs between present and future satisfactions. But then the third stage of what had been a long developed relationship between psychology and economics saw the systematic attempt to completely eliminate psychological content from economics. Why?—Just after the year 1900 there was great dismay among economists over a new development in psychology that was not amenable to any interpretation as (economic) utility maximization. The great dismay at that time, among all of economics, was due to the theory of unconscious motivation that was published in Freud's *Interpretation of Dreams* (1901).

So I ask you to just think about what we have here historically. In the mid-1750s Adam Smith is worried that reason, combined with human frailty, can lead to destructive interpersonal conflict. And then 150 years later, we might say that Freud comes along and shows us that reason, combined with human frailty, can lead to destructive in*tra*-personal conflict.

It is only most recently, 100 years after Freud's mark, that economics and especially behavioral and cognitive psychology applications to economics are admitting that their greatest challenges lie ahead. And these challenges, they now claim, are to discover the *deeper secrets* of the wealth of nations; the faculties that Adam Smith called our moral sentiments or what it is about human nature that we call humane.

Unfortunately, thus far, anything psychoanalytic remains banished from the theoretical approaches that are being brought to get at these "deeper secrets". The 250 year evolution of the economic and behavioral economic theory that began with Adam Smith and the social matrix through which it operates is almost phylogenic in its nature and its repressive structure. *The basic assumption is that humans can be represented as homo economicus and that all behavior can be represented as one-dimensional motivation. This is what all of the MBA's in our corporations have been taught in their graduate educations for at least the past half century.*

So finally now, perhaps we have arrived at a time when there has been enough gone amuck, repeatedly, in management and policy and corporate governance that psychologists of economics say we must get at "deeper secrets". At least the idea of *deeper* has broken through the repression barrier. Unfortunately what they all want to do is "relax the assumptions" of the 250-year-old structure around the rational model but still get all of us to aim for the perfection of rationality. Or as a recent *New Yorker* article (Cassidy 2006) on neuroeconomics reported, several studies include MRI's and brain scans to observe our internal warring sides under stress and the effect of this on the brain. Still, in spite of referring to internal warring sides, which means that on some level there is recognition of human ambivalence, not a word about psychoanalytic or psychodynamic.

So having put you through this digression, frankly with the purpose that you might begin to feel the repressive weight of this dysfunctional view that has trained our corporate managers, I will dare to offer a psychoanalytic perspective on this impulse toward "deeper secrets" that we here all realize does exist within homo-economicus. And this perspective will parallel the nature of the corporate conundrum.

The opening phase of any psychoanalysis, after all, is usually the person realizing that his or her own self interpretive system is breaking down. And by the way, ladies and gentlemen, recall that in early November 2008, we watched Alan Greenspan a bit shaken when he admitted before a congressional committee that the efficient economic paradigm he had so idealized he now realized had been wrong, even though many Nobel Prizes had been given for this particular economic ideology.

The good news here is that paradoxically the impulse towards a depth of understanding always comes at the moment that one "can't understand". So now our greatest hope and the psychoanalytic way in to the economic organization dilemma should be that we grasp that even behavioral economics "doesn't understand"; that is, that it doesn't get at human depth and that mechanically it cannot.

So with the ubiquitous nature of corporate fraud that we believe we realize, let's think about what happens inside organizations if stock prices, for example, become dramatically wrong; especially if the prices are *over* valued. And equity is over valued if the management team cannot deliver the performance that the market requires to justify its stock price. This sets up powerful organizational forces that can lead to the destruction of value. One financial scholar, Michael Jensen (2004), who is emeritus at Harvard, suspects that the phenomenon is almost like organizational heroin and all the managers contribute. When the process with overvaluation begins it feels good for the management. But then, like the effect when one tries to get off an addiction from drugs there will be extreme human pain down the road.

If the equity is really overvalued it begins to dawn on top management that they have a big job to justify the price. On the other hand, overvalued equity is cheap currency in acquisitions. Banks make it easy for the organization to get debt if there is equity as yet unrecognized as overvalued. Such a circumstance will have managers doing things that they would not otherwise do, such as overpay for acquisitions, hence destroying value in the company. These actions also lead to destroying earning which then begins to affect operations. As the pain down the road begins to set in, after the earlier high that felt good becomes harder to sustain, managers who have been honest and are otherwise honest people may be driven to push the numbers in such a way that is a walk around the corner to fraudulent reporting.

After all there is not likely to be the appropriate listening by the Board of Directors in the early stages of overvaluation. The CEO can't often go to a Board and say "we have to eliminate our overvaluation". The Board will not likely be happy to hear it. CEO's end up flogging organizations for 40 percent annual growth and it becomes like pouring gasoline on a fire. The Board didn't want to hear about overvaluation. Organizations cannot rely on capital markets to solve the problem because the markets have been part of its systemic nature. Eventually after that turn to fraud has happened the problem falls back on some sort of corporate governance system, albeit too late if at all.

Some five or six years ago there was a study done by academician, Renee Stulz and two colleagues. Their results were titled "Wealth Destruction on a Massive Scale" (Moeller, S., Schlingerman, S., & Stulz, R.M. 2005). What their data showed was that in the 1990s, acquiring firms lost $240 billion dollars of value around the announcement of mergers. This was compared to $4.2 billion loss of value of acquiring firms in the 1980s. They cite for the 1990s an average loss of $2.31 per $1.00 spent on acquisitions. Management may be able to con the market for awhile but then the market sees through the incredible plunge. The pressure of the anxiety within organizations is tremendous. They are trapped in the reciprocal impact of psychic and systemic factors on their ability to implement new approaches. United in a mutual craziness people go through as-if operations.

So while major organizational change efforts should almost be the more constant norm in today's environment to avoid the kind of vulnerability to fraud that we now see; it will require structural conditions within firms in order to adequately contain the profound anxieties that are experienced via repetitive upheaval. And by the way, the Behavioral Decision people, if we psychoanalysts learn to communicate with them, could help us here. But in the absence of improved conditions that will help to contain anxieties, change efforts are likely to fail because managers and employees will both turn to destructive defenses in order to protect themselves. The wish for change seems accompanied by its opposite and delusional aspects may arise in any of us whereby there is no way to integrate contradictory wishes. These defensive mechanisms can make conflicts within our minds impossible to own. And we cannot analyze what is not there.

At some level it all comes down to processing anxiety whether your system shuts down or becomes an occasion for an opening of the new and hopefully a new symbolic meaning that will help to interrupt the omnipotence of overvalued equity in anything: stocks, houses, etc.

And by the way, if you recall one of the remarks from Smith's *Moral Sentiments* that I mentioned: that happiness has to do with the consciousness of being beloved

Well, Freud believed that maturity of being able to integrate opposing emotions (love and hate) is one of the things that make us lovable.

What psychoanalysis has to offer our thinking, and research, and management and hopefully even economic policy-in-the-sky, is ways to open up the space of anxiety and to come in to the gain of capacities that we didn't have before.

It is NOT just about exchanging equity/debt, merger, acquisitions, etc. *It is about being able to create conditions that will help sustain anxiety so that we can open new human capacities.*

So how can psychoanalytic theory begin to show the economic world that it has something to offer this quest for understanding "deeper secrets" of humankind?

My hope is that we can begin to provide research that will use a principle that remains a cornerstone of our psychoanalytic thought – and that is the postulate that belongs to psychoanalysis; the postulate of *ambivalence*. The nature of ambivalence offers two enhancements to the 250-year development of the certainty of the rational aim.

First: the nature of ambivalence is to hold opposing affective orientations toward the same person or object. This is a phenomenon that does not lend itself to elegant mathematical models. And second: rational aims have remained attractive as the singular aims in theoretical support because they are regarded as being relatively stable. Ambivalence on the other hand tends to be unstable, expressing itself in different and sometimes contradictory ways as actors cope with it (Smelser 1998).

And although ambivalence differs from the idea of the rational my argument for progress at getting to deeper secrets is this: the notion of ambivalence leads us to understand and explain a range of behaviors and situations beyond the scope of rational choice explanations however far the "rational" may be relaxed or stretched.

Who knows? Maybe psychoanalysis can begin to change the phylogenic structure of the hold that economics and the behavioral segment of it have had on insisting on man's univalent condition, remember now, for 250 years.

If we think about it all of these troubled firms in the news seduced others into believing one could master the social fantasies that fuel the market. Mathematical modeling does not fuel the market. Mathematical modeling is a fantasy of mastering the fantasy structure of capitalism. The idea that you can have capitalism without risk or that every loss/panic can be converted into gain/excitement is really the ultimate (potentially fascist?) fantasy.

I believe that we psychoanalytic thinkers can help economics to get to the "deeper secrets" what Adam Smith was seeking about the humane in an integrative way. Of course we will challenge the power and the omnipotent greed that economics has been unable to relinquish for so long.

REFERENCES

Arrow, K., Yew-Kwang, N., & Xiaokai, Y., eds. (1998). *Increasing Returns and Economic Analyses.* New York: Palgrave Macmillan.

Cassidy, J. (2006). What Neuroeconomics Tells Us About Money and the Brain. *The New Yorker,* Septermber 18.

Freud, S. (1899–1901). The Interpretation of Dreams. *Standard Edition,* Vols. 4 and 5.

Jensen, M. (2004). from remarks made at: "A Conference in Honor of Finance Professor Eugene Fama," May, 2004, University of Chicago Booth School of Business.

Moeller, S., Schlingerman, S., & Stulz, R.M. (2005). A Study of Acquiring-Firm Returns in the Recent Merger Wave. *Journal of Finance* 60(2):757–782.

Smelser, N. (1998). The Rational and the Ambivalent in the Social Services. *American Sociological Review* 63:1–16.

Smith, A. (1759). *The Theory of Moral Sentiments.* Original published in Scotland; Amherst, NY: Prometheus Books, January 2000.

——— (1776). *An Inquiry into the Nature and Causes of the Wealth of Nations*. Chicago: University Of Chicago Press (facsimile of 1904 ed. edition), February 1977.

Leslie Shaw, Ph.D.
980 North Michigan (#1400)
Chicago, IL 60611
Leslie@leslieshaw.com

Bryant Welch

CHAPTER 8

State of Confusion: Assault on the American Mind

I don't want to just end the war;
I want to end the mindset that got us into war.
—Barack Obama

America is rapidly becoming a nation psychologically unable to confront its problems. From the White House, from the media, and from the pulpit, Americans have been deceived by predatory political forces into fighting a disastrous war, squandering our national wealth, destroying our standing with other nations, and neglecting badly needed initiatives at home. It is a series of failures that will haunt America for generations to come. And it will not end simply because George Bush has left office.

America has been gaslighted. Gaslighting is an insidious set of psychological manipulations that undermine the mental stability of its victims. These techniques have invaded our media, infiltrated our churches, and attacked our most basic free institutions. Sadly it has even infected the American Psychological Association as APA's recent tragic response to the Bush Administration's detention centers has shown. For millions of Americans the techniques have altered the way they think, feel, and act. It has been nothing less than an assault on the American mind.

I am a clinical psychologist and attorney. I have spent half of my thirty-year career treating patients in intensive psychotherapy. The other half I spent in Washington, D.C., much of it in a political position with the American Psychological Association. There I had the opportunity to study politics, politicians, and political manipulation firsthand as few clinical psychologists have.

My recent book *State of Confusion: Political Manipulation and the Assault on the American Mind* (2008) explains from a psychological

---

This article originally appeared in *Psychologist-Psychoanalyst,* the newsletter of Division [39] of Psychoanalysis of the American Psychological Association, Vol. XXVIII, No. 3 (Summer 2008), pp. 6–10.

perspective how and why these manipulative and destructive techniques are now deeply imbedded in our political system and why they are having a progressively debilitating effect on the American mind. If Americans do not recognize them and confront them, the country will be less and less able to respond rationally to the very real crises facing us. And if we psychologist-psychoanalysts do not help America do that, who will?

Why have Americans become so vulnerable to divisive political tactics? *Why* did America get dragged into such an unwise war in Iraq? *Why* do fundamentalist religious groups, Fox News, and right-wing hate radio now play such influential roles in America's political landscape? *Why* are long-accepted scientific ideas like evolution under siege? These questions, and others, puzzle people from all points on the American political spectrum and from all points around the world. *What has happened to the American mind?*

The term "gaslighting" comes from the 1944 movie *Gaslight,* starring Charles Boyer and Ingrid Bergman, in which a psychopathic husband, coveting his wife's property, tries to drive his dependent young bride insane by covertly manipulating her environment, leaving her increasingly perplexed and uncertain. Among other things, he raises and lowers the gaslights in the house while denying to the wife that there has been any change in the lighting. He feigns genuine concern for her, but cleverly isolates her from any contact with the rest of the world, as a result of which she might become independent of his propaganda-like assault on her sense of reality. He fires the trusted elderly maid and replaces her with a younger one whom he can seductively control and who is naturally competitive with his young wife.

With a combination of seduction, deception, isolation, and bullying, he so warps his wife's reality-sense that she gradually begins to accept his "reluctant" suggestion that she is losing her mind. She becomes almost totally dependent upon the husband to tell her what is real and what is not real in spite of periodic clues that he is lying and really quite hostile and hateful towards her. Just as she is on the brink of a complete nervous breakdown, a perceptive Scotland Yard detective who has become suspicious of the husband and uncovers his machinations, rescues her. When he exposes the husband's deceptions to the wife, she regains her stability and is able to confront her husband forcefully as he is taken off to jail.

For many of us in the mental health profession, the term "gaslighting" refers to a series of mind games that prey on our limited ability to tolerate much ambiguity or uncertainty about what is truly happening in important areas of our lives. It is a highly destructive form of psychological manipulation that undercuts one's trust in one's sense of reality and results in confusion, perplexity and an inability to make sense of one's world In the search for a resolution to their bewilderment people often become extremely vulnerable and dependent on someone else whom they regard as omniscient and to whom they look to "clarify" confusing events. This makes them vulnerable to manipulators and false prophets. This is what has been inflicted on large segments of America.

Throughout my seventeen years in Washington, DC, I lobbied and managed myriad psychologically-related issues in the public arena. I am proud that during those years, the APA was in the forefront in addressing important issues such as the recognition of the rights of sexual minorities, the need to address psychological trauma as a consequence of war and disaster, and the need for a truly national health care plan. As an attorney, I also fought against large (Health Management Organizations (HMOs) in courtrooms around the country on behalf of mental health patients who had suffered the all-too-often fatal effects of our current system of managed health care.

When I moved to Washington to enter the political world, I was initially struck by the contrasts between our clinical work and political work. In the treatment setting, two people are working as hard as they can to achieve greater self-understanding for the patient. This requires tremendous candor. In the political world, in contrast, smoke and mirrors predominate and are often weapons of choice. In therapy people are searching for their true motivations; in politics they are often trying to obscure them.

But, ultimately, the experience that I brought from the therapeutic consulting room to the Washington political world was invaluable. I began to see that transcending that difference between the political world and the therapy world was the human mind, working the same in both the clinical and the political settings. Psychological concepts such as "resistance," "symbols," and "transference" were extremely helpful in learning how to develop a political legislative campaign. Understanding and being able to read the nature and depth of certain emotional states, like envy and narcissism, helped avoid pitfalls that could invite political opposition from the people whose support we badly needed.

At first I thought using these psychological tools was just the only way *I*, given my background, could make sense of politics. With time, I concluded it was the only way politics *does* make sense.

But there was another part of the psychological world in Washington for which I was not so prepared. There is a widely known and very old saying in Washington, "If you want a friend, get a dog." That is an overstatement, but not by as much as one might think. And the reason for that is because Washington is a beehive of deception where one can never be sure of what is real and what is not real. Who is sincere and who is just very good at pretending to be sincere? It can get very confusing. In Washington, gaslighting reigns.

I saw many individuals painfully gaslighted in work and organizational settings. I saw whole organizations undercut by manipulative CEOs. But when gaslighting is done to an entire country as it has been to the United States, the results are chilling. In America the political use of gaslighting is leading to a psychologically impaired and unstable American electorate. The resulting policy decisions that are made have devastating implications for all Americans and for the world.

Once Americans adopt the irrational beliefs and become dependent on the gaslighter, they are highly unlikely to reconsider their beliefs no matter what the consequences and no matter what the evidence to the contrary. This is why it was so easy to adjust the rationale for the Iraq war retroactively so many times. With remarkable ease, America's cause went from eliminating weapons of mass destruction to evicting an evil dictator, to spreading democracy, because the idea that our leaders might have been wrong, incompetent, or worse was simply too disconcerting a proposition for many Americans to consider. An already traumatized and confused nation, bombarded by messages from people on whom they had become increasingly dependent, was simply too weak to rebel.

But why is there such dependency? As we all know, a fundamental aspect of human psychology is the mind's effort, its outright *need,* to have a reality of which it feels certain The reality it creates may or may not be accurate. That is less important. From the point of personal psychological need, it is better to *feel* certain than to *be* right. The mind simply cannot function well without this certainty and, if it feels uncertain, it will seize on almost anything for help. This is the pressure point of maximum vulnerability in the human mind, a point that right-wing ideologues have long known how to press—and that progressive liberal forces are only now beginning to address American politics is now a battle to shape what Americans perceive as reality.

Making *reality* a political battleground means that in America reality is up for grabs, and the long-term risk is that voters will become the prey of anyone who seems to provide security, strength and certainty.

When a persons, or a nations, sense of reality is repeatedly manipulated by clever people with devious intent, the victims' ability to function effectively is eroded and he or she becomes disoriented. Rationality falls by the wayside. People, and nations, behave erratically and because of ever-increasing uncertainty, become dependent upon demagogues and ideologues that speak confidently and appear to offer escape from confusion This has happened to millions of Americans who, often lured by moralists' bromides, have turned to neo-conservative spokesmen, ministers, and politicians and become dependent on them, even enthralled by them.

It is remarkable how many of these prominent political and religious spokesmen to whom conservative Americans have looked for help, have themselves been exposed for serious hypocrisy, preaching morality but practicing what they themselves have labeled immorality. What is even more astonishing, however, is how dependent and willing to overlook hypocrisy and deception millions of their followers are. *This reluctance to see the gaslighters for what they are is the cornerstone of the gaslighting relationship.*

In March 2007 former House Speaker Newt Gingrich, shortly after publishing his new book, *Rediscovering God in America* (2006), admitted that he was having an affair with a younger employee at the same time he was leading the impeachment of President Clinton for not being forthcoming about the same offense. Gingrich had the chutzpah to imply that his willingness to risk being exposed as a hypocrite at the time of the impeachment was a profile in political courage. But this same allegation of hypocrisy could just as easily be attributed to Rush Limbaugh, William Bennett, Rev. Ted Haggard, and Bill O'Reilly all of whom were caught in the most remarkable scandals for individuals assuming their self-righteous postures of moral superiority. With the exception of Haggard, none appears to have suffered any lasting effects.

In the movie *Gaslight,* the gaslighting husband fired the elderly maid and carefully controlled any outside influences that threatened his own control of his wife's reality sense. Similarly, today's gaslighters have extended their reach throughout American society in multiple ways to increasingly control the information Americans receive about the world. They have invented a 24-hour-a-day, 7-day-a-week cable pseudo-news channel, co-opted evangelical religious leaders, and viciously attacked their opposition with smear campaigns and lies.

At the same time, professions that have historically played important roles in helping us define our political reality are all under attack—mainstream media, law, education, even science, have all suffered a precipitous decline in influence. Thus, the American mind is on the one hand assaulted by powerful new forms of deception and, on the other, abandoned by institutions that have traditionally been supportive of independent, liberal thought. Given the complexity of our present situation, this could not have occurred at a more unfortunate time.

In America today, psychological gaslighting exploits people already confused and perplexed about an increasingly complex world. Leaders are deliberately misleading them making their world more confusing and making them struggle with explosive, but only subliminally recognized, psychological states. The current assault on the American mind is taking place because of three specific, emotionally-charged psychological states: paranoia, sexual perplexity, and envy. These are the true "battleground states" in American politics today. Whoever carries the day in addressing and harnessing these psychological states will control and shape the American political landscape for the coming decades. Any political party or movement that fails to consider them in its camaign strategy will be significantly handicapped. That party may win under certain circumstances but the odds are heavily stacked against it.

The genie cannot be put back in the bottle. The methods of gaslighting are now deeply and permanently ensconced in our political system and will not go away. The forces are there, the techniques operative. Unless we learn about these techniques, and how to defend against them we will continue to suffer from them. But when we do understand how the mind works—how certain states of mind affect us in our political behavior—it provides us with a powerful and consistent explanation for America's behavior in today's political world.

American politics, now and for the future, will be the politics of reality. Any party that does not try to articulate a reality that appreciates the needs and complexities of the human mind will become increasingly obsolete. For a nation armed with nuclear weapons to suffer the psychologically-regressive effects of gaslighting at the same time it is grappling with the post-9/11 loss of its island-fortress security is a highly combustible combination that is terrifying in its potential consequences. *State of Confusion* is my attempt to sound an alarm to these dangers, describe the psychological dynamics behind them, and suggest potential remedies to prevent their potentially devastating consequences.

An understanding of the human mind is the key tool of the new political architect and psychologist–psychoanalysts more than any other professionals have the understanding to explain and make constructive use of those tools. Thus, it was not surprising that it was APA Division 39 (Psychoanalysis) that was the most articulate and vociferous opponent of the American Psychological's recent shocking support for the Bush Administration's "enhanced interrogations" at detention centers around the world. It is a tragic case study that occurred very close to home.

Why Did the APA Do It?

The regressive effects of gaslighting have taken their toll on the psychologists' national organization, the American Psychological Association (APA) as well as our country. Many mental health professionals were shocked when APA three times refused to take an unequivocal stance against psychologists' participation in the Bush detention centers. The fact that other health care organizations, typically more conservative than APA on humanitarian issues, were very outspoken about the issue made it all the more puzzling.

In human rights groups and liberal organizations around the world the arguments APA spokespersons advanced in support of APA's position did not pass the red face test for credibility. Instead, their seemingly transparent disingenuousness only made psychology sound embarrassingly like the Bush Administration.

Banning psychologists' participation in reputed torture mills was clearly unnecessary, it was argued. To do so would be an insult to military psychologists everywhere. Psychologists would never engage in torture. Further, psychologists' participation in these detention centers was really an antidote to torture since psychologists' presence could protect the potential torture victims. We were both too good and too important to join our professional colleagues in taking an absolutist moral position against one of the most shameful eras in our country's history.

There are two questions that beg for answers. How did the APA form such an obviously close connection to the military? And why did the APA governance—the Board of Directors and the Council of Representatives—go along with the military interests? How could an organization of such bright people be rendered so incompetent to protect the profession from the horrible black eye they have given us?

I have had ample opportunity to observe both the inner workings of the APA and the personalities and organizational vicissitudes that have affected it over the last two decades. With one interruption, for most of the twenty- year period from 1983 through 2003, I either worked inside the APA central office as the first Executive Director of the APA Practice Directorate or served in governance positions including Chair of the APA Board of Professional Affairs and member of the APA Council of Representatives.

When the torture issue broke last year, the answer to the first question about APA's military connection seemed obvious. Since the early 1980s, APA has had a unique relationship with Hawaii Senator Daniel Inouye's office. Inouye, for much of that time, has served as Chair of the Subcommittee on Defense for the Senate Appropriations Committee. The Subcommittee has responsibility for all U.S. defense spending. One of Inouye's administrative assistants, psychologist Patrick DeLeon, has long been active in the APA and served a term as APA president. For over twenty-five years, relationships between APA and the Department of Defense (DOD) have been strongly encouraged and closely coordinated by Dr. DeLeon. It was DeLeon acting on behalf of Inouye who initiated the DOD psychologist prescription demonstration project in the late 1980s that began psychology's efforts to secure prescriptive privileges.

For many APA governance members, most of whom have little Washington political experience, DeLeon is perceived as a canny politician and political force on Capitol Hill. The two most visible APA Presidents on the torture issue, Drs Ronald Levant and Gerald Koocher, based on personal discussions I have had with them in recent years, clearly hold DeLeon's political savvy in high regard.

While I personally got along well with DeLeon and never doubted his commitment to psychology, his view of psychology and his sense of priorities were quite different from mine, and I did not share the assessments of DeLeon's political prowess. I felt his priorities had more to do with the status of psychology as reflected in comparatively minor issues that were often unconnected to issues that were of true importance to practitioners. Rightly or wrongly, I often felt that an accurate sense of context was missing from his political analysis and objectives. It's the same feeling I have now when I look aghast at what APA has done on the torture issue. Except this time, it is not something relatively innocuous.

Some people attempt to explain APA's recent seemingly inexplicable behavior by assuming that large sums of money changed hands on the torture issue. I could certainly be wrong, but I think the more likely (and more remarkable) explanation is that the judgment of those making the decisions was simply that bad and that insensitive to the realities of the human suffering they were endorsing.

Regardless, there is no question that APA had formed a strong relationship with military psychologists and the DOD through its connections with Inouye's office. But it is the second question that is probably more difficult to understand from afar. How could both the APA Board of Directors and the APA Council of Representatives support the military on this issue and subject the profession to such embarrassment by supporting a policy that is anathema to the vast majority of psychologists?

Here's how. The pluralistic and multifaceted governing process that I saw when I entered the APA in the early 1980s ended in the 1990s. Differences of opinion stopped and the APA suffered a terrible regression. Increasingly inbred under the administration of APA President Dr. Raymond Fowler, the association agenda was primarily financial, focusing on making money both through real estate and through what many of us felt was unwarranted, financially harsh treatment of APA employees.

More peculiarly, Fowler's "agenda" for APA was encapsulated in the phrase "working together" a noble idea that, to the best of my knowledge, was never attached to any actual substantive agenda. Instead, it served as a means of social control, a subtle injunction against raising any of the conflictual issues, challenges, or ideas that need to be addressed in any vital and accountable organization.

The result was that much Council intercourse turned into fawning over one another. Many members appeared to me to bathe in the good feeling that came from "working together." For some, the bath was a narcissistic one and organizational regression became more debilitating. In other instances during this period, dissent by rank and file members was stifled with heavy-handed letters from the APA attorney threatening legal action or communications from prominent members of the governance threatening ethical action if policy protests were not discontinued.

As a result of the regression, the governance of APA was ill prepared for thoughtful deliberation on a matter as important as the torture issue. As I have written in *State of Confusion,* when people are confused, they are eager to be told what is real. The governance was simply over its head in trying to deliberate effectively on such an issue when there was organized support on the other side coming from the military interests and the upper echelon of APA leadership like Drs. Koocher and Levant.

When the torture issue arose, the Council, despite the efforts of Division 39 members, fell victim to some of the very silly arguments described above. Council members were told that to oppose psychologists participation in the detention actions was to suggest that our colleagues might engage in torture. In a fashion chillingly characteristic of the gaslighter (described above), it was implied that those who raised concern about torture, were themselves torturing their colleagues who were working in the military. One prominent member of the APA governance gratuitously raised the ethnicity of one of the military psychologists, seemingly opening the possibility that the opponents to torture were racist.

These arguments were then followed with the grandiose closing argument that psychologists presence at the detention centers was critical to make sure torture did not recur. We psychologists had a moral duty to prevent immoral behavior. The piano player, once aroused to the possibility of what was going on upstairs, was now needed to prevent it. Yes, these were the arguments that carried the day in APA deliberations. In the more discerning eyes of the world, they have very little credibility.

But the gaslighting is not over, even now. Ultimately in a remarkable display of activism by APA members, they expressed the will of the membership by banning psychologist participation in the detention centers. At present, the measure has been in effect for over a year, but the ruling elite at APA has disputed this and failed to implement the will of the members. Who rules APA? Its members or the military? Despite being an organization of psychologists, APA has been subjected to very little analysis.[1]

RERERENCES

GINGRICH, N. (2006). *Rediscovering God in America: Reflections on the Role of Faith in Our Nation's History.* Nashville, TN:Thomas Neslon.

OBAMA, B. (2008). quotation from January 31, 2008 Presidential debate with Sen. Hillary Rodham Clinton ("I don't want to just end the war . . . I want to end the mindset that got us into war.")

WELCH, B.(2008). *State of Confusion: Political Manipulation and the Assault on the American Mind.* New York: Thomas Dunne Books.

END NOTE

1. For an update on the analysis of the American Psychological Association, see blog by Bryant Welch: "Torture, Psychology, and Daniel Inouye: The True Story Behind Psychology's Role in Torture." *Huffington Post,* June 16, 2009.

Bryant Welch, J.D., Ph.D.
19 Shelter Cove Ln Ste 204.
Hilton Head Island, SC 29928
E-mail: welchfirm@aol.com

Peter Wolson

CHAPTER 9

Political Power: An Alluring Stimulant for Regression and Omnipotence

"Power tends to corrupt, and absolute power corrupts absolutely." Most of us are familiar with the first sentence, but few know the sentence that follows: "Great men are almost always bad men," said Lord Acton in 1887, in a letter to Bishop Mandell Creighton (1904). Political power often appears to be a stimulus for regression to primitive dynamics, characterized by grandiosity and omnipotence. Under its intoxicating influence, one can easily slip into feeling like, "His majesty, the baby," as Freud (1914) put it, entitled to have anything heart, stomach or loins desire. Greed prevails!

Just think of the politicians who have acted as if the laws of civilization did not apply to them—Nixon wiretapping those on his "enemies list" and breaking into the Democratic Party's national headquarters at the Watergate Hotel to steal political information; JFK frolicking with prostitutes in the White House pool (Hersch 1997), Clinton pardoning fugitive Mark Rich putatively? in exchange for contributions to the Clinton Library; George W. Bush torturing detainees at Abu Ghraib and Guantanamo in violation of the Geneva Conventions Senator Stevens taking bribes and calling them gifts, and Governor Palin attempting to have the Wasilla librarian to remove books which offended Palin's religious beliefs; New York's Governor Spitzer's rendezvous with prostitutes and Illinois Governor Blagojevich's. attempt to sell Obama's vacated Senate seat. Often these politicians transgressed in the full light of day. without shame or guilt.

It is like the fable of the Emperor exhibiting himself naked in what he believed to be his new clothes, projecting his grandiose self-deception into his subjects who were blinded or too intimidated by their fear-induced idolatry totell him the truth. Only a child, insulated from this pathological idealization could see his nakedness and point it out.

The danger of regression to omnipotence in heads of state has been intuitively recognized for centuries. Thus, the crucial role of the king's court jester. Only the "royal fool" had the right to speak the truth and poke fun at the king, bursting his grandiose bubble without risking his life. The devalued status of "the fool" permitted the king not to take the blows to his omnipotence seriously, which minimized his humiliation and narcissistic rage. The jester kept him grounded in reality.

It is therefore not surprising that many of America's founding fathers were extremely relieved when George Washington refused to become the King of America, and participated in designing a constitution with checks and balances to limit the potential abuse of the Chief Executive's power. America has struggled with the Presidential inclination to abuse power ever since.

Psychologically, how does political power induce regression to omnipotence? Freud (1914) theorized that all of us begin life totally self-absorbed, in a state of primary narcissism. As infants, we lack the cognitive and perceptual capacities to distinguish ourselves from the outside world. Nothing exists apart from our selves. Thus, we begin life feeling omnipotent, like God. We are motivated by our immediate impulses and exploit our parents to fulfill our needs. Greed predominates and we feel entitled to have whatever we want. When frustrated, we become enraged and want to destroy the source of frustration.

Through parental discipline, socialization and psychological maturation, we gradually learn that we are not omnipotent, that we need to depend on others for vital caretaking. Our parents help us respect others, modulate our aggression and differentiate right from wrong, especially through a healthy resolution of the Oedipus complex. But, according to Freud (1914), we all pay a heavy psychological toll for repressing our infantile narcissistic longings. We lose our pre-Oedipal paradise in which we felt that the world was our oyster, in which we could demand the satisfaction of our immediate impulses and, in fantasy, wreak the most horrific vengeance, against those who defy us. Throughout life we are burdened by constantly having to suppress these unconscious, primitive impulses.

The experience of political power is ominously similar to our infantile experience of "His majesty the baby,“ Nothing could quite equal the euphoric experience of fetal "enwombment" or early infancy when all our needs were taken care of and we were under the sway of our delusions of magical power. When our mothers carried us down the street, total strangers stopped to lavish praise upon us and tell us how cute we were. It was downhill after that. As we grew older, we had to work harder and harder for less and less attention and reward. No wonder psychoanalysts have emphasized the pervasive human urge to regress, to return to early childhood where we can once again be the center of our own universe with our intoxicating feelings of omnipotence. The power, celebrity and attention that comes with high political office often trigger these repressed longings and the propensity to regress to infantile dynamics. It is, therefore, not surprising that many politicians have narcissistic trends in their characters, especially adaptive grandiosity.? Originally, I related adaptive grandiosity to artistic creativity, as "the individual's exhilarating conviction of his potential for greatness, the extremely high value he places on the uniqueness of his feelings, perceptions, sensations, memories, thoughts and experiences" (Wolson 1995). "It is an ego-state which can be conscious or unconscious. This clearly differs from normal healthy self-confidence in which an individual believes in the value of his perceptions and in his capacity for successful achievement, but lacks the pervasive grandiose qualities described above" (Wolson 1995). Adaptive grandiosity is inextricably intertwined with reality testing, with secondary process thinking and with the separation of the self from others. As a result, behavior emanating from this ego-state is reality- oriented and adaptive. For the artist, adaptive grandiosity was deemed necessary to help overcome separation anxiety when confronting the blank canvas. Similarly, adaptive grandiosity in politics provides the motivational fuel to step into the unknown, to take creative risks as a political leader and to exert one's energy, intelligence and fortitude often against insuperable odds. This was evident in J.F.K's proposal of a space flight to the moon, and the intense application of his ego-strength to achieve this goal. It is evident that Barack Obama's willingness to venture into the ambiguous terrain of , our devastating economic and military crises. is that he has a grandiose conviction of his wisdom and ability to find a solution. Many pundits were awed by Obama's unusual aplomb and audacity in facing these challenges that would bring most self-confident people to their knees.

The concept of adaptive grandiosity is an extreme manifestation of healthy narcissism, and is most similar to Kohut's concept (1971) of the archaic grandiose and idealizing selves as necessary building blocks for ambition, goals, and achievement. However, it is also a manic defense against the politician's depressive reaction to separation from the maternal introject when having to step into the void as a leader and confront the unknown.

Because of its fragile nature as a manic defense, adaptive grandiosity can easily regress to maladaptive grandiosity, in other words, omnipotence: a belief in magical control of both external and internal objects, an inclination toward fusion states, an inability to distinguish between self and other and the euphoric feeling that one can do or have whatever one wants, regardless of human limitations. During the political process with its intoxicating fame, adulation and power, the politician's adaptive grandiosity often yields to the temptation of regressing to infantile dynamics and omnipotence, unleashing Pandora's box of greed in all of its manifestations.

Psychoanalytically, Gordon Gekko from the movie, *Wall Street* (1987) was, to some degree, right. He said, "Greed is good. . . . It is the essence of the evolutionary spirit. Greed, in all of its forms—for life, for money, for love and for knowledge—motivates the upward surge of mankind". The Kleinians, for example, would argue that greed is the basis of love and dependency, epitomized by the baby's urge to consume the breast. If one regards greed as the baby's primordial lust for life and the oral foundation of our psychosexual longings for control, money, sex and knowledge, it is a powerful source of motivation for achievement and fulfillment in all aspects of human endeavor. However, for this to be so, it needs to be contained and regulated by ego-strength, which is inherent in the dynamics of adaptive grandiosity. In contrast, the uncontained greed that is triggered by omnipotence is often destructive and self-destructive. We saw this in Illinois Governor Rod Blagojevich's impeachment following his unrealistic demand to head a foundation supported by Bill Gates and Warren Buffet as one among many requirements in exchange for his nomination of an Illinois Senator to replace Barack Obama. With maladaptive grandiosity, the emperor believes that he should be appreciated in his new clothes, or as Nixon said in the movie, *Frost/Nixon* (2008). "When the President does it, it's not illegal;" or, President Clinton's grandiose belief that he could have oral sex with Monica while on the phone conducting a war in the Balkans, not considering how this might impede his judgment or impair his legacy. And, of course, he was impeached for perjury, obstruction of justice and abuse of power because of his relationship with Lewinsky and the Paula Jones lawsuit.

Adaptive grandiosity may be the outcome of excessive adulation by a mother, which will undermine the complete separation of the self from the object, and reinforces archaic grandiosity (Wolson 1995). Moreover, there is probably only a partial resolution of the Oedipus complex; some crucial identification with the paternal object remains to form the final ego ideal. Such identifications facilitate the connection between grandiosity and secondary process functioning. Chasseguet Smirgel (1984) said that achieving identification with the paternal object helps the child separate from the primary fusion with mother and is a major developmental step toward separation-individuation. This step represents a change from the pleasure principle to the reality principle, and from primary process thinking to secondary process thinking" (Wolson, 1995). To the extent that excessive primary narcissism continues to prevail and that a positive Oedipal resolution is not fully achieved, with the ego-ideal partially merged with the ego, the person becomes the embodiment of his or her own ideals. This results in a grandiose confidence in one's capacity, and an extremely high sense of personal self-worth. Moreover, the person has reached a sufficient level of individuation, and object relatedness along with the full use of secondary process functioning. This provides an extraordinary capacity for success.. The regression of adaptive grandiosity to omnipotence depends on the strength of secondary process functioning. The greater the person's ego-strength, the less likely the regression.

A good illustration of adaptive grandiosity versus maladaptive grandiosity is a comparison of Barack Obama with John McCain in the recent 2008 presidential election campaign. Obama appeared to be extremely determined, well-measured, energetic, and exceptionally self-confident as he organized what is considered the best campaign in presidential election history. And of course, he is an eloquent, charismatic speaker. His success seemed to be fueled by adaptive grandiosity. The prominence of his grandiosity was evident in the Al Smith roast in which he poked fun at his own arrogance and sense of "specialness," David Brooks, the New York Times columnist, quoted an item in The New Yorker on the Chris Mathews show. The item said that Obama had the chutzpah to tell an aide, ("I know more about speech writing than my speechwriters, I know more about policy than my policy directors and I think I know more about politics than my political directors." Thus, there was some basis for McCain's campaign mocking him as "the chosen one," and criticizing him as too ambitious McCain displayed adaptive grandiosity in his remarkable perseverance especially in the face of fairly certain defeat. However, in contrast to Obama's calm and thoughtful determination, he was erratic and impulsive, desperately flinging mud at Obama and making grandiose but empty gestures. For example, during the congressional bailout talks, he temporarily suspended his campaign and rushed to Washington, as if riding in on a white horse to save the day. But he was marginalized, even by fellow Republicans, and rendered impotent. The main theme of his campaign was self-aggrandizement. "Elect me because I am great, I am experienced, I am a war hero." And yet what we saw was an impatient, immature politician grandstanding and losing emotional control.

His friends and political colleagues were shocked. They said this wasn't the John McCain they knew, possibly the Senator most skilled and remarkably effective promoting and passing difficult legislation. We witnessed this John McCain immediately after his defeat in the graceful, admirable concession speech he delivered.

Apparently, his maladaptive grandiosity was triggered when he finally won the Republican nomination for the Presidency. Everyone observed McCain regress before his or her eyes into "his majesty the baby," the anti-authoritarian maverick. The adaptive grandiosity that helped him get elected to the Senate and contributed to his stellar career had disintegrated into infantile narcissism characterized by impulsivity and lapses in judgment and integrity.

In effect, he regressed to his former impetuous self when he was an anti-authoritarian "hot-head," a player, carousing with the ladies and an impulsive daredevil who crashed planes during his naval training, oblivious to the cost to the American taxpayer.

According to his biographer, John McCain had been the apple of his mother's eye. She raised him single-handedly while his father; a four-star Admiral, was largely absent and emotionally distant. At puberty, McCain changed from a quiet, obedient, courteous boy into a mischievous rebel. In high school he was nicknamed "Punk" and "McNasty" by his peers (Timberg 1995).

Psychologically, he seemed to be struggling with a conflict between the demanding superegos of his father and grandfather that required duty, service, conscientiousness and adherence to a stellar military tradition and his rage against being controlled by paternal authority. Until his POW experience he felt that he had failed to fulfill his father's expectations, This history appears to reflect a partial Oedipal victory and paternal abandonment resulting in adaptive grandiosity and a predilection for defiance.

John McCain said that his Vietnamese POW experience motivated him to dedicate his life to his country rather than to personal gratification. His many productive years in the Senate reflected this dedication.

Unfortunately, under the alluring influence of the political power he acquired by winning the Republican nomination for President, he regressed.

In contrast, Barack Obama committed only a few narcissistically devaluing faux pas during the campaign. These included his devaluing depiction of blue-collar workers in Western Pennsylvania as bitterly clinging to guns and religion due to job losses, and, shortly after winning the election, his contemptuous remark about Nancy Reagan conducting séances. For the most part, he was exceptionally careful and calm in the face of all the mud that was hurled at him, reflecting excellent secondary process functioning. His ego-strength limited his potential for regressing to maladaptive grandiosity.

Similar to McCain, Obama was largely raised by mother figures: his grandmother and, to a lesser degree, his mother. The latter essentially abandoned him for philanthropic pursuits. His father divorced his mother and returned to Kenya when Obama was two.. One might infer that he also had a partial Oedipal victory with some positive male influences through his Indonesian stepfather, who taught him to fight, and through his grandfather who adored him. However, at ten, Obama finally met his real father for a few months and was extremely impressed with his charismatic eloquence and mesmerizing storytelling, as were his mother and grandparents. As a young adult, Obama learned that his father had returned to Kenya and soon became financially successful working for an oil company. Having political aspirations, the elder Obama worked for the Department of Finance and rose to become a senior economist. But he was outspoken against government corruption and offended Jomo Kenyatta, Kenya's President. He was subsequently fired, blacklisted, and could only obtain a low-status job in the water department. He turned to alcohol, became impoverished and died in a car accident

In this history, we see the psychogenic basis of Obama's adaptive grandiosity, his partial Oedipal victory, the male influences of his stepfather, grandfather and his idealized real father who was eloquent, inspirational and had his own political ambitions. The title of Obama's autobiography, *Dreams From My Father* (1995), displayed reflected this ego-ideal. Obama had a confusing, detached, lonely childhood, moving from Hawaii, to Indonesia, to Kansas. During late adolescence he drifted toward drugs, alcohol and depression, but his grandmother confronted him about the importance of respecting himself and applying his intelligence and talents to create a good life. He took her admonitions to heart and credits her and the influence of his mother (Meacham, 2008) for his success.

In addition, he was confused about his identity, raised by whites while being half black and looking black. It wasn't until he was in college and began to immerse himself in black culture that he finally consolidated his identity and felt at home. He seems to have projected his longing to repair his fragmented self-structure onto the political landscape with his sublimated aspiration of unifying the disparate, compartmentalized, multicultural, multiracial, multi-political aspects of American society. His newfound political power has not yet triggered a regression to infantile dynamics.

In contrast, the regression to maladaptive grandiosity was paramount in the "imperial presidency" of George W. Bush, as the Los Angeles Times (Editorial, 2008) termed it. As Republican Governor of Texas, George W. was known as a conciliator with the Democratic power blocs in the State Senate and House of Representatives. Based on his track record, he justifiably ran for President as a "compassionate conservative," which appealed to many voters who knew of his ability to make compromises with his political opponents. The major contradiction to this picture was his lack of compassion in commuting sentences for convicts appealing their death sentences. He rarely commuted a sentence, even when presented with new evidence indicating an incorrect conviction. As the ultimate arbiter of justice, he was a hanging governor. He seemed to believe that sticking to his guns, regardless of guilt or innocence, was strong, and reversing the court order would be weak. This rigid attitude foreshadowed his presidential masculine bravado.

Shortly after becoming President and sustaining considerable media criticism for his mispronunciation of words and lack of intellectual gravitas, George W was saved by 9/11. Strutting with a macho swagger, he became one of the most grandiose, omnipotent Presidents in American history, the "war president," as he put it. This display of maladaptive grandiosity seemed, in part, to be a way of compensating for his profound sense of inadequacy. In an Op-Ed article for Counterpunch, I demonstrated how the Bush regime displayed all the symptoms of a narcissistic personality disorder.

A narcissistic display of grandiosity usually compensates for a sense of vulnerability and helplessness. Clearly, 9/11 made Americans feel extremely vulnerable and, consequently, perhaps, willing to accept President Bush's grandiose policy of unilateral preemption without much protest. Years before 9/11, the neo-cons Richard Perl and Secretary of Defense Paul Wolfowitz expressed the belief that the United States, as the most powerful country on earth, has the right to remove forcibly the leaders of other nations who are judged to pose a threat to American security, and to impose a democratic form of Government upon them. As President Bush recently told Tim Russert on Meet the Press, he reserves the right to wage war to achieve these goals without having to consult with the international community. The Bush administration's grandiosity was also demonstrated in the mistaken belief that the Iraqis, after thousands of years of living under authoritarian governance, would heartily welcome the American liberators and the chance to establish a democracy. Instead, American soldiers were generally greeted with resentment and terrorist attacks. The anticipation of a joyous welcome was a narcissistic projection of the Bush administration's idealized, egocentric belief system and reflected a lack of empathy for a different culture.

"A narcissistic personality fears dependency which will make him feel weak, humiliated and dominated by the other. In an increasingly interdependent socio-economic world, the Bush administration seems to have feared that involvement with other countries would threaten the United States in danger of being controlled and exploited by them. The antipathy to participation in the United Nations and even NATO was an attempt to defend America against this vulnerable, dependent position.

The narcissist demonstrates a dominating, exploitative use of others, and an inclination to use or ignore the law if it interferes with his goal.. It appeared that the Bush administration would engage with other nations only when it was dominant and able to use them for to attain its own goals.. Thus, it was willing to ask other countries for soldiers and equipment, as long as it could retain control, rather than share the decision-making power in rebuilding, Iraq. Amore mature form of international collaboration would have been the sharing of power and responsibility on an egalitarian, mutually respectful basis."

The grandiose idealization of "going it alone," certainly appeals to the American West tradition of rugged individualism. But when taken to the extreme of a lone gunslinger, fighting the "evildoers" who are "wanted dead or alive," it smacks of defensive grandiosity. As a result of its isolationism, the Bush administration had to face the responsibility of American soldiers dying from terrorist attacks daily with few international troops for support. The narcissist is convinced that it is "a dog-eat-dog world," one can only trust one's self, and has a predilection for "splendid isolation," to use Kernberg's (1975) term. "Since dependency is psychologically dangerous, the only one the narcissist can trust is himself." The Bush Administration seemed to believe that the United States could rely only upon itself. The guiding principle of unilateral preemption is: "Do unto others before they can do unto you." Thus, this was the rationale for President Bush's preemptive attack against an "imminently threatening" Saddam Hussein.

In addition, the ability to award lucrative contracts to Halliburton Co. in which both the Bush and Cheney families have had financial interests, raises questions of self-serving.

What was the genetic basis of George W's ostensible regression to maladaptive grandiosity? This regression was fueled by primitive dynamics. Because his father was away for considerable periods of time engaged in business and politics, George W. grew up more closely involved with his mother (Minutaglio 2001). But at as early as eight years of age he demonstrated a precocious ability to work the room during his father's campaigns, hobnobbing with prospective benefactors and soliciting their support. This was an early sign of his enormous confidence in his ability to win over adults through his social charm and personality, perhaps the pre-eminent feature of his "good ole boy" rise to the Presidency. Nonetheless, his younger brother, Jeb Bush, the past Florida Governor, revealed that George W. felt the pressure of living up to his father's example. As analysts, we know that when the father is extraordinary or inaccessible, or a combination of both, as was George H.W., the son's idealization can increase monumentally, which makes it harder to believe he can ever match his father's achievements.

Brothers Jeb and George W. referred to their father as the "beacon" (Minutaglio 2001) also George W. was intimidated by his father's disapproval. Barbara Bush explained her husband's disciplinary method: "The way George scolded was by silence or by saying, 'I'm disappointed in you.' And they [his sons] would almost faint." According the younger brother Marvin Bush , George W's. reaction to his father's words was extreme. would be made to feel that he had committed the worst crime in history. When 19-year-old George W. quit working on an inland barge seven days before his job commitment was to end, his father said, "I just want you to know that you have disappointed me." George W. ran out of his office and has said he remembered those words for years.

George W. believed his father was superior to most men at whatever he did. The son's academic and work history virtually replicated his father's, but, in many instances George W. fell short of his father's accomplishments. He was a cheerleader at Yale, not a star baseball player.

He was in the Navy reserves ducking a Vietnam War assignment, not a war hero, and he failed at multiple business enterprises, which his wealthy family financed. His underachievement could well have been a reaction to the pressure he experienced trying to live up to his father's image.(Wolson 1999).

It seems that George W. might have unconsciously coped with his critical super-ego through alcoholism and an anti-authoritarian mischief-making and rabble-rousing. During his father's 1988 presidential campaign, according to George W. commented it would be better for him if his father lost the election and retired to private life because of the enormous expectations for a son in politics whose father was president. (Minutaglio 2001).

George W.'s transformation from an impulsive alcoholic to a serious politician seemed to be a result of his wife's influence and of his religious conversion. He came to believe that God wanted him to be President and was guiding his destiny. This projection of omnipotence into God served both adaptive and maladaptive functions. Adaptive grandiosity impelled by religious zealotry, motivated him to control his impulsivity and employ his social skills and cunning to win the Governorship of Texas and the Presidency.

However, once he became President, his regression to infantile dynamics and omnipotence became palpable. How much of George W.'s God-inspired "macho" grandiosity as in invading Iraq and toppling Saddam was fueled by an Oedipal defiance and a wish to triumph over an idealized but castrating internal father? He all but declared that his father had failed to complete the job in the first Iraq war. By rejecting the counsel of his father's trusted advisor and friend, James Baker, and his father's policy of international negotiation in favor of a policy of American domination, it was as if he tried to prove that his father was the castrated male, not himself.

Clearly, political power can be a dangerous inducement to the tyranny of primordial impulses over reason. And these impulses and infantile dynamics can be transferred through projective identification into a nation's psyche, as seemed to occur in the administrations of George W., Richard Nixon and in the Russian Government of Joseph Stalin.

Stalin is obviously an extreme example of adaptive and maladaptive grandiosity. Under the influence of his adaptive grandiosity, the Soviet Union became one of the two most powerful nations on earth, but Russian society became as paranoid as Stalin (Montefiore 2003). His regression to omnipotence was so profound that he gradually expected his political cohorts to read his mind, as if they were primitively merged with him. They knew that if they failed to do so, they could be sent to the gulag and/or killed. Moreover, Stalin induced a culture of omnipotent gratification among his henchman. For example, Beria, head of the secret police, allegedly a good family man, felt the sadistic entitlement to pick up any woman he desired and rape her. In some cases, he exploited her by promising to free their husbands from the gulag, but after gratifying himself, failed to honor his promises.

Stalin was an abused child, beaten daily by his drunken father. He was favored by an adoring mother, who was also an alcoholic and often beat him. In order to protect himself, he retreated to his room and read all the books he could gain access: philosophy, history, literature, and economics. Like many successful narcissistic personalities, he had numerous talents and skills. As an adolescent, a number of his romantic, lyrical poems were published and became minor Georgian classics. He sang so well in the church choir that he was considered good enough to become a professional; He was also a talented painter. However, the Russian revolution became his greatest passion and he raised money by becoming a bank robber and a murderer (Montefiore 2007).

On a number of occasions, he was arrested and exiled to live with families in remote areas of Russia. Inevitably, he would seduce the wife and/or daughters of the household, but was so charming and intimidating that the husbands outwardly accepted these trespasses. Lenin picked Stalin as a co-leader of the revolution because he wanted a bloody revolution and knew that Stalin was a killer (Montefiore 2003).

Clearly, Stalin suffered from malignant narcissism; he was paranoid and a sociopath. Unlike most sociopaths, however, he could control his impulses. An interesting side-note was his idealized identification with Adolph Hitler, a malignant twin ship of brothers in evil (Montefiore 2003). This fraternal bond was cemented in Stalin's psyche when he learned of Hitler's "Night of the Long Knives," in which the latter had the SS murder the members of the SA, who had been his most loyal supporters and enforcers. He apparently feared that the SA was acquiring too much power. Stalin thought this a brilliant strategy, and seemed to emulate it with many of his closest associates, eventually having them imprisoned and/or killed.

His fraternal bond with Hitler was consecrated with the Molotov-Ribbentrop non-aggression pact in the early stages of World War II.

When his advisors informed him that Hitler was on the verge of invading Russia and bombing Moscow, he couldn't believe it. He imprisoned the messenger and protested repeatedly that this wasn't possible. When the bombs fell on Moscow, he was dazed and confused, clinging to his delusion that this was merely a provocation by Hitler. Stalin's defense ministerswere paralyzed, fearful of provoking his ire. But he quickly reconstituted and devised a brilliant strategy which ultimately defeated the German army.

Toward the end of his administration, Stalin retreated to an isolated dacha and complained that nobody wanted to visit him, possibly re-enacting his lonely childhood and exile in Siberia. However, he commanded his chief ministers to attend monthly late-evening feasts which extended into the morning at which he forced them to consume great quantities of the most delicious food available while the rest of Russia starved. He would require them to eat and drink beyond their capacity until they regurgitated and were totally inebriated. He would then exhort them to consume anew, while he monopolized their attention with repetitive recitations of his youthful exploits long into the night. Bored nearly senseless, drunk and bloated, they mustered all their willpower to look attentive. They would inevitably begin to fight with one another while he listened very closely for any signs of betrayal. History demonstrates how , political power can easily trigger regression to maladaptive grandiosity and destructive greed. Our hope with the new administration is that Obama's grandiosity remains adaptively fueling his creativity in resolving the complex, daunting problems facing America today and not regress to omnipotence and greed. Like every king, he needs the equivalent of a court jester. He gets these from Saturday Night Live, late-night T.V comedians, journalists and political pundits, and the confrontation by his powerful team of strong-minded individuals. As with any political leader, we need to remember Lord Acton's profound, but chilling insight, "Great men are almost always bad men" (Creighton 1904).

REFERENCES

CHASSEGUET-SMIRGEL, J. (1984). *Creativity and Perversion.* New York: W.W. Norton & Company.

CREIGHTON, L. (1904) *The Life and Letters of Mandell Creighton.* D.D. Oxon and Cambridge, Volumes 1, 2.

FREUD S. (1914). On Narcissism. *Standard Edition* London: Hogarth Press, 1957.

HERSCH, S. (1997). *The Dark Side of Camelot.* New York: Little, Brown & Co.

KERNBERG, O. (1975). *Borderline Conditions and Pathological Narcissism.* New York: Jason Aronson, Inc.

KOHUT, H. (1971). *Analysis of the Self.* New York: International Universities Press.

MEACHAM, J. (2008). On His Own. *Newsweek. (*September 1st, 2008 issue*).*

MINUTAGLIO, B. (2001). *First Son: George W. Bush and the Bush Family Dynasty.* New York: Three Rivers Press.

MONTEFIORE, S. (2003). *Stalin: Court of the Red Tsar.* New York: Vintage Books.

——— (2007). *Young Stalin.* New York: Alfred A. Knopf.

NEWTON, J. (2008). Editorial: Obama's Victory is a Mandate for Change. *Los Angeles Times.* (November 5, 2008).

OBAMA, B. (1995). *Dreams from My Father.* New York: Times Books.

TIMBERG, R. (1995). *John McCain: An American Odyssey.* New York: Free Press.

WOLSON, P. (1995). The Vital Role of Adaptive Grandiosity in Artistic Creativity. *Psychoanalytic Review*, 82, 577-597.

——— (1999). When Politics is also Psychology. *Los Angeles Times "Opinion" Section.* (12/5/99).

——— (2004a). Politics of Narcissism: America's Grandiose Persona Under Bush. *Counterpunch*, (February 14/15)

——— (2004b). The Underlying Dynamic of Post-9/11 America: Exhibitionistic Revenge at Abu Ghraib. *Counterpunch*, (May 22/23).

Peter Wolson
450 North Bedford Drive (#301)
Beverley Hills, CA 90210–4307
Peterwolson@earthlink.net

Mitchell Wilson

CHAPTER 10

Greed Wrap-Up, or Gift-Wrapped Greed

My intention in these remarks is to take what you've heard from our psychoanalytic presenters over these past two days, and, with the help of psychoanalytic theory, integrate some of their ideas into a narrative.

I'm going to emphasize the following interlocking points: (1) the dead seriousness of greed; (2) its independence from usual symbolic and oedipal relations; (3) its visual aspect and that the greedy person is caught in a scenario; (4) the status of the desired object; (5) the role of the father; (6) issues of triangulation, the analytic third, and bias. This last topic—bias—will takes us rather easily into our final panel in which considerations of the psychology of decision-making and its impact on investments with be discussed.

First: greed is remarkably unfunny. Now you may immediately reply: "Wait. Jeff Stern was funny." And Jeff was. He was funny because he took an ironic distance from his subject—Eliot Spitzer. Certainly we feel a kind of Schadenfreude experience at the great falls of the truly greedy. That is from the outside looking in. From the inside, from the subjective experience of the greedy themselves, it's not a pretty picture. From this first person point of view, there is nothing foolish, funny, or whimsical about greed. As Arlene Kramer Richards stresses in her paper on gambling, there is a "furious seriousness" at work here—a ferocity about all serious attempts at avariciousness, at covetousness. Several contributors to this volume make a distinction between wealth creation and greed. Wealth gets mixed reviews, but greed, in the end, is one big sack of woe.

There is an important sense in which greed doesn't fit into our usual psychoanalytic theory. That is, there is nothing in it of the old Freudian *witz*, the humor of the unconscious, the way conflict and compromise show themselves in the Vanity Fair that is life—the kind of thing that lends itself to "making fun of," including, most importantly, the making fun of oneself.

Greed is different. Scrooge isn't funny. Charles Boyer's Gregory in *Gaslight* (1944) isn't funny. Zasu Pitts's Trina in Von Stroheim's classic film *Greed* (1924) is not either. Ken Lay? Bernie Madoff? Eliot Spitzer? You get the idea.

Why is this? Greed seems to live in that split off place that is outside the conventional symbolic order, by which I mean the usual set of social relations in which we all engage. These social relations are based on some sense of the Law, in which one has to compromise, negotiate, tell the truth (at least most of the time), and struggle with disappointment and loss. If it is true that greed resists the symbolic order, it is also true that greed fully partakes in the relatively unmediated, visual order—what Jacques Lacan (1977a) calls the "Imaginary." Notice that the root of the word "speculator" is the Latin *specere*, "to look." Let's consider Zasu Pitts as Trina in the aforementioned movie *Greed*. Pitts masterfully uses her rapacious eyes (they seem to take over her entire face) to signify her equally capacious appetite—a kind of visual hunger that—as Jeff Stern and Bob Galatzer-Levy both suggest, is an *un-conflicted* hunger. Trina's hunger is un-conflicted because her super-ego, her moral center, is not involved. Pitts' Trina is not caught up in the normal pushes and pulls of desire, which involve necessarily a relationship to the Law. And as both Stern and Galatzer-Levy make clear, because greed is split-off it is filled with anguished excitement, fear, and quiet desperation. Charles Boyer in *Gaslight*, also, like Pitts, uses his eyes to express a single minded mania for jewels; at other times, as you can see in this scene with Ingrid Bergman, he uses them to manipulate the reality of his unsuspecting wife.

It is of crucial importance to see that the greedy are caught in a coercive scenario—a scripted scene that is autonomous, independent from the world around it, and in which the greedy character is *con*-scripted. The object of visual interest—gold and jewels—looks back at the subject as if absolutely controlling his or her every movement. In this sense the greedy are objects of something larger than themselves. Trina will hold onto her gold coins in perpetuity no matter what misfortunes befall her. Gregory's actions appear to be less endlessly repetitive than Trina's, but have the same relentless ferocity. As Gregory says at one point: "Jewels are wonderful things. They have a life of their own." The Latin origin of "speculate" helps us again: a *specule* is a "watch tower." Hence the feeling of claustrophobia, scripted internment, subtle paranoia, and hopelessness that emanates, like an effluvium, from those caught in the unwavering, repetitive nature of their actions.

Several of our contributors emphasize the driven quality, the desperate repetitiveness, of these scenarios of greedy action. They stress the key ingredient of omnipotent fantasy as a motivating force of the greedy. But notice but that the omnipotence is *virtual*—as is most omnipotence. The greedy person fools himself into thinking he's in total control; yet, he's feeding a beast that controls him. Envy is always a scripted scenario in just the way I am describing—the envious person covets that which he thinks he wants, all the while being ruled by envy, and controlled by its object. Destroying the envied object—ruining and spoiling it—always involves a kind of self-ruining, a self-destruction.

In these discussions, it is tempting to imagine that only *some* egregious souls are plagued by greed and envy, and we are not they. Of course, the fact is that all of us have a place in our minds that is not dissimilar from the dynamics our presenters attribute to the famously greedy.

Another important aspect of greed is that it is often based on a lie. As opposed to conflicted actions that are mixtures of desire and guilt—what Kohut (1971) called Tragic Man—the truly greedy are fraudulent and fully aware of it. They don't lie to themselves; they lie to others. In other words, the economy of *self*-deception with which all of us deal—the ways we find out, often after the fact, that we've lied to ourselves—does not seem to apply to the truly greedy. As Jeff Stern writes in his imagined analysis of Eliot Spitzer, there were two Spitzers. The Eliot that frequented his DC prostitute was fully aware that he was doing it, and presumably was fully aware that he was not coming clean to his wife. Trina, in *Greed*, is fully aware that her starving husband is pounding the bitter streets of San Francisco, struggling to scrounge two bits together to buy a can of beans, while she is in bed night after night fingering, and sleeping with, her gold coins.

Which leads us to another key aspect of greed, one that Janice Lieberman and Bob Galatzer-Levy emphasize. This is the peculiar status of the *seemingly* desired object—that which the greedy person *appears* to desire. Let's look at Trina again, because in her relationship to her gold coins one finds something essential, something basic in the very structure of greed. As the movie unfolds, after a while you realize that this woman has no intention of spending her money. As her and her husband's fortune declines, she holds onto those coins, fingering them sensuously, laying with them. The coins have ceased to be money in the sense of something to be exchanged for something else. They are simply fetishized objects, rock-solid in their emptiness. They stage a *fundamental impossibility*: she cannot spend the coins because then they would cease to be the fetish-objects she needs them to be. If spent, they would take on a certain value and meaning—they would represent, for example, food or clothing—they would enter the world of exchange—the Symbolic—which we infer would be much too much for her to handle. They would cease to be the concrete, meaningless objects she needs them to be. Like a hamster caught on a wheel, Trina's desire is dead—she is lost in a repetitive, driven scenario. One gets the distinct sense she is better off with her coins. What we learn is that the object of desire is never really *it*; it just *seems* to be it.

Our contributors emphasize a point that is directly related to this issue of a kind of "reluctance" or refusal to enter into the Symbolic order. In the "biographies of greed" of which they write, they place much emphasis on the role of the father. Either the father is overly present, narcissistic, and controlling, like Eliot Spitzer's, or he is distant and self-involved, like the fathers of George W. Bush and John McCain. (Notice that the distant father exerts another kind of power, of course, in relation to the idealizing child.) Or as was the case in the Barthelme brothers' gambling fiasco, the father is dead. This reminds of me of the epigraph to Donald Barthelme's novel of the same name: *The Dead Father* (1975). The epigraph reads: "The Dead Father is a motherfucker." The dead father is such a one if he has not been properly mourned, if he has not, as it were, been properly buried. The Barthelme brothers' relationship to their father seems to reveal a need to "settle accounts"—to even out the balance sheet. One can only conclude they felt, unconsciously, that they owed their father a debt that had to be paid by their gambling away their inheritance.

The essential point here is one that both Peter Wolson and Richard Tuch stress: that if you have a complicated or faulty identification with the father, then you will have great difficulty entering the symbolic order. The father can be neither too close nor too distant—if he is either then his presence is traumatic: the son is objectified and can't *have* the father in the psychoanalytic sense of using the object (Winnicott, 1969). The father can't be used symbolically—the son cannot identify with his function. In other words, if the child cannot relate to the father in a meaningful way over time, then the father can't separated *from*. Janice Lieberman's description of her clinical work with certain extremely affluent patients points us in the same direction. These patients, having been prevented from learning from life experiences, prevented from risking and at times failing, lack a kind of "fiber," the emotional strength to make their way in the world. Instead, they tend to be overly dependent on their parents, and manipulate reality to hide this dependency from themselves. They are also, as Janice describes, very difficult to engage in treatment, since the therapy can so easily become yet another aspect of the disavowed realities that mark these patients' lives.

In psychoanalysis this symbolic father and the law he represents has taken on other contemporary meanings. I have in mind the "analytic third" (Ogden, 1994). Many analysts have described certain key elements that are crucial to the development of a solid analytic process. These include that the analyst does not work simply from a "knowing" position in relation to the patient, making assertions about the patient's internal life and attributing mental states to the patient; nor does the analyst work naively in a "relational" field, as if both parties are equal and there are no differences between them. There must be a point of reference outside the dual relation of the patient-analyst pair that gives *perspective* on the process, that *orders* what would otherwise be an imaginary, phenomenological experience (Wilson 2003). This third is usually conceptualized as the unconscious—that which is *other* to the prevailing, more conscious discourse. Dreams, slips of the tongue, enactments—such are some manifestations of the "analytic third." The psychoanalytic point, though, is that the symbolic father is the ancestor or predecessor to this third. Bryant Welch, in his paper on Gaslighting, makes it clear that without a third term, a perspective, hypothesis testing is impossible—that is, the testing of one's ideas against reality is very difficult. In the movie *Gaslight* (1944), Ingrid Bergman is in a dual relationship with Gregory, her husband. Gregory limits his wife's exposure to the outside, so she is unable to test her sense of things. The detective, played by Joseph Cotton, is precisely that third term which allows perspective and reality to give her mind shape and help her to figure out what is really going on.

This issue of perspective, of the third, of the father, brings me to my final point, and will serve as a segue to the final panel of papers. Several of our contributors discuss the psychological aspects of decision-making at length. Leslie Shaw's entire paper is devoted to ways in which economic theory has, over its intellectual history, first ignored psychology, then gradually embraced it, but in a form—cognitive science—that has left it, from her point of view, conceptually bankrupt. This conceptual bankruptcy is because there is a resistance in economics to modeling ambivalence and conflict. Part of what Leslie writes can lead easily enough into a question—a question that psychoanalysis as a field of knowledge has continually struggled to answer—that is, the question of how psychoanalytic knowledge gets out into the world and is used in other fields. The problem is, as Leslie says, that analytic ideas are routinely ignored by other disciplines, especially in the social sciences. Worse than this, analytic concepts are not only ignored but are often smuggled into economic and psychological models and called by other names. No doubt, this bothersome fact has something to do with the relative and self–imposed isolation of psychoanalytic institutes from major centers of learning, our research universities.

As I said, this is a major topic and one I will not venture into further except to tell one brief anecdote. I happened to meet George Akerlof, the Berkeley professor who won the Nobel-Prize for economics a few years back for his work on asymmetric information (Akerlof, 1970). He told me he was writing a book on "identity" and economic decision-making. He wanted to know if what he was writing rang true from a psychoanalytic point of view and asked me to take a look at a draft of the book. In the book Akerlof and his co-author Rachel Kranton (2010) attempt to include what he calls an "identity utility" into the standard economic model; that is, to account for an individual's preference for group identification as a motivating factor in how a person spends his/ her/ their time and money. Often, Akerlof claims, people spend money in the "name" of something, even though there is no "material" benefit. Though Erik Erickson's (1950) work on identity, and Jacques Lacan's (1977b) work on symbolic identification and the crucial difference between symbolic value and biological need—though these ideas are used throughout Akerlof and Scranton's book, they were not identified with psychoanalysis nor was specific credit was give to Erickson and Lacan. Analysts such as Erickson and Lacan were working on these ideas sixty years ago. It is as if they were whispering in the wind and no one was listening, except a few psychoanalysts huddled close together in a small corner of the intellectual landscape.

The issue of perspective, or what analyst's call the "third," is directly related to what psychologists such as Kahneman and Tversky (see Tversky, 2004) discovered in their work on judgment and decision-making under uncertain conditions. What they discovered is known as *confirmatory bias*. The vast influence of their work is well-known to many of you. I like to think of it as entirely consistent with what analysts have understood since Freud (1901) wrote in Chapter 7 of the *Interpretation of Dreams* on hallucinatory wish fulfillment, and continued with in

On Narcissism (1914)—that *thinking is inherently wishful*. This means that all assessment and judgment—no matter how "rational"—is shot through with a self-preservative, self-aggrandizing investment. Confirmatory bias means that we want to confirm our current assessment of a situation. Sometimes this is called *status-quo bias*. First impressions, as economists Rabin and Schrag (1999) have shown, often *persist* in the face of contrary evidence, and may get *solidified* in the face of more and more contrary evidence. Reference levels, risk-aversion, assessments of similarity, over-valuing small sample sizes (the power of "low numbers"), not taking into account the prior probability of the likelihood of the thing under consideration to actually happen—all of these facts about the mind support and extend what analysts have long-known about the narcissistic basis of thinking. Though analysts may have known this, we have often forgotten it, or repressed it, because for a long time analysts did not like taking uncertainty and bias into account. This is why the analytic third as a concept has come to the fore, and why analysts can always benefit from ongoing supervision, study groups, and the like, because all of us work under the constant threat of narcissistic closure.

The crucial issue of confirmatory bias is directly related to the subject of the final series of papers: gullibility and investing.

REFERENCES

AKERLOF, GEORGE A. (1970). The Market for 'Lemons': Quality Uncertainty and the Market Mechanism. *The Quarterly Journal of Economics*. 84:3, pp. 488–500.

AKERLOF, G.A. & Kranton, R.E. (2010). *Identity Economics: How Our Identities Shape Our Work, Wages, and Well-Being*. Princeton, NJ: Princeton University Press.

ERIKSON, E.H. (1950). *Childhood and Society*. New York: Norton.

FREUD, S. (1899–1901) The Interpretation of Dreams, *Standard Edition*, Vol. 4 and 5.

——— (1914) On Narcissism. *Standard Edition*, 14:73–107.

KOHUT, H. (1971). *The Analysis of the Self: A Systematic Approach to the Psychological Treatment of Narcissistic Personality Disorders*. Monograph Series of the Psychoanalytic Study of the Child Monograph No. 4. London: Hogarth Press; New York: International Universities Press.

LACAN, J. (1977a). The Mirror Stage as Formative of the Function of the I as revealed in Psychoanalytic Experience. in *Écrits: A Selection*. Transl. Alan Sheridan. London: Tavistock, pp. 1–7.

——— (1977b). The Function and Field of Speech and Language in

Psychoanalysis, in *Écrits: A Selection*. Trans. by Alan Sheridan. New York: W.W. Norton.

OGDEN, T.H. (1994). The Analytic Third: Working with Intersubjective Clinical Facts. *International Journal of Psychoanalysis*. 75:3–19.

RABIN, M. & SCHRAG, J.L. (1999). First Impressions Matter: A Model of Confirmatory Bias. *The Quarterly Journal of Economics*, February.

TVERSKY, A. (2004). *Preference, Belief, and Similarity: Selected Writings*, ed. Eldar Shafir. Cambridge, MA: The MIT Press.

WILSON, M. (2003). The Analyst's Desire and the Problem of Narcissistic Resistances. *Journal of the American Psychoanalytic Association* 51:71–99.

WINNICOTT, D.W. (1969). The use of an object. *International Journal of Psychoanalysis* 50:711–716.

Mitchell Wilson
2960 Piedmont Avenue
Berkeley, CA 94705
E-mail: mdwmd@comcast.net

Symposium 2009 Sunday Panel Presentations and Discussion

Stephen Greenspan, PhD
Consulting Psychologist and Author,
Littleton, CO

I am pleased to chair the session on "Investor Gullibility." Our panel consists of three presenters who are authorities on investor risk assessment and a discussant who is an authority on psychoanalytic theory. I am an authority on neither, so it is reasonable to ask, "how did I come to chair this session?" So I will start off this session by answering that question, before turning the floor over to the others.

I had been laboring for over two years on a book titled *Annals of Gullibility* (Greenspan, 2008). On December 10, 2008 I held the first copy in my hands. On December 12, I learned that Bernard Madoff had swindled a chunk of my retirement funds. Finding this too amazing to keep to myself, I wrote a lengthy article for *Skeptic* magazine's website, and it was reprinted as a featured weekend essay in the *Wall Street Journal*. As might be expected, it received a lot of attention, including from the organizers of this conference.

Some of the attention reflected, undoubtedly, the ironic aspect of my situation. For example, one blogger in Canada wrote, "the first Greenspan, Alan, will be remembered as the former Fed chairman who didn't see it coming, while the other Greenspan, Stephen, will be remembered as the gullibility expert who forgot to read his own book." This irony struck many people as funny, and certainly reinforced the idea that anybody, even an authority on gullibility, is capable of being gulled. Of course, my interest in gullibility reflects in part my own past experiences with the phenomenon. Knowing about gullibility has probably made me less gullible than in the past, but all human beings not living alone in a cave are always at risk of being seriously duped.

More than this irony of a gullibility expert being gulled, I think my article on investor gullibility struck a nerve because its analytic framework, borrowed from my book, was seen as answering fairly well a puzzling question, namely "how could so many intelligent investors have made the seemingly unintelligent decision to turn over much (in some cases, all) of their fortune to a swindler?" I used this framework to explain human financial vulnerability, relying on a case illustration I knew quite well, namely myself. In fact, it was a very appropriate illustration to use, because all four of the factors in my explanatory framework played a role in my own foolish behavior.

My theory of human gullibility can be considered broadly psychodynamic (in which case my participation in this conference may be appropriate after all). It bears some similarity to Freud's structural model, in that any foolish (or nonfoolish) act is seen as resulting from the interaction of three within-person forces intersecting with a situational challenge. (I see gullibility as a sub-type of a broader class of "foolish"—i.e., risky—behaviors, as described in Greenspan, 2008). The three within-person forces are "cognition" (analogous to ego), "personality" (analogous to superego) and "affect/state" (analogous to id). The situational challenge in the case of gullibility is the inducement to behave foolishly (i.e., to see a risky situation as safe) that results from persuasive pressure by one or more other people.

The external aspect, which I term "situations" is the first of the four factors in my explanatory model. It is ever-present in all Ponzi schemes and investment manias, as described by Robert Shiller (2006) in his book *Irrational Exuberance*. It applied in my own case, in that my decision to invest in the Rye/Tremont hedge fund (the second largest of the Madoff "feeder funds") was impelled by my exposure to a group of investors in South Florida—and their highly-trusted adviser—who all extolled the virtues and safety of the fund's slow but steady annual returns.

The second factor in my model (and the first of the within-person factors) I term "cognition." It refers to the amount of knowledge and expertise one possesses in a particular content area. I know little about hedge funds and lacked the expertise to independently assess the risks associated with the investment. This made me more susceptible to social pressures than would otherwise have been the case.

The third factor (and the second within-person factor) I term "personality." It refers to one's degree of interpersonal trust and one's inclination to look deeply into a potentially risky decision. I happen to be very high on interpersonal trust and very prone to impulsively take risks without a lot of reflection. These are not good traits to possess when crossing paths with a skilled con artist.

The fourth factor (and the third within-person factor) I term "affect/state." It refers to any self-regulatory imbalance that acts as a motivating force. This could take the form of affect (fear, greed), which increases the attractions of a particular course of action, or state (exhaustion, inebriation), which reduces one's ability to resist those attractions. In my own case, and that of most Madoff victims, affect played an important role. Specifically, the affect took the form of excitement and relief at having found what appeared to be the perfect long-term investment instrument during a time of great financial uncertainty.

Most cases of foolish investing can be understood, I believe, to result from the confluence of these four factors: exposure to a persuasive investment scheme, relative inability to recognize the risks in that scheme, unwillingness to seek more information about those risks, and excitement about the promised benefits of participating in the scheme. In my own case, all four factors played an equal role. In other cases, one or two factors may have played a predominant role (as in the case of relatively knowledgeable investors whose critical faculties were hijacked by affectively-driven self-deception processes). I am confident that the remaining four presentations will provide useful information about the phenomenon of investor gullibility, the adequacy of my explanatory theory, and the precautions that investors can take when exposed to deceptively attractive investment schemes.

Christopher J. Topolewski, Esq.
Investment Advisor, West Capital Management
Philadelphia, PA

What I am going to speak to you about today are cases that come directly from my firm, West Capital Management. West Capital Management is a wealth management firm whose people work very closely with our clients. We believe that working this closely with them gives us an understanding into their thought process, how the clients analyze different investments, and what really leads them to their final decisions. And it is this close working relationship that we believe we have with clients that is a reason why Chris Cutler of Management Analysis Services asked me to come today to speak about our experiences with several of our clients. The examples that I will describe involve very smart people who are our clients. They have had very successful practices and they have run very successful businesses themselves. But what I will walk you through in the examples is that the clients' skills in their own successful businesses did not translate into being good investors and being able to make a rational decision when it came to actual decisions with regard to their own money and their own finances. So even though a lot of what we do is portfolio construction as a wealth management firm, another part of our role is helping to keep our clients out of trouble and avoiding bad strategies. And today I have two examples for you.

The first example involves a company called "Classic Star." Classic Star was (and actually it is still in existence) a company that was based in the State of Kentucky. The Classic Star strategy was to help medical professionals, sports athletes; and other kinds of business owners reclassify their income from what was received in their actual professions claiming the revenue from a different income category that would be in the category of "agricultural."

Now this does sound very strange at first. And the strangeness of this income re-classification strategy is probably the first warning sign. {Laughter} But the reason for wanting the income re-classification to agriculture is very appealing. The appeal comes from many prior years during which time Congress has helped the American farmer with varieties of tax credits in order to smooth the cyclical nature of the farming business. Crops have good years and bad years. In order to help smooth out taxes, Congress has devised varieties of tax credits for farmers. And if it is possible to have your income categorized as agricultural, you will have tremendous tax benefits.

As it turned out there were several West Capital Management clients who were in medical practice together and the group known as Classic Star approached them. A very elaborate promotional tour was arranged for our clients. They flew us from Philadelphia in a private plane down to Kentucky. We had box seats at the Kentucky Derby. There were elaborate spreads, there were celebrity endorsements. There were sports figures there who were actual clients of Classic Star and who also endorsed the deal. The structure of the deal, essentially, was that Classic Star would help you set up your own farm in Kentucky. Our clients supposedly would then lease mares, the female horses, from Classic Star for breeding purposes. The clients would also, via Classic Star, be raising young foals and foaling into being one year and two year horses and then sell them at auction. So that is the way that the Classic Star strategy was supposed to work.

When we came back to Philadelphia our firm, West Capital, actually retained two different CPA firms to determine legitimacy of the deal.

Neither of them could establish how we could reclassify a doctor's practice as agricultural. And West Capital also did background on the due diligence of the Chicago law firm that had supplied an opinion letter for Classic Star. That is to say an opinion letter where the law firm says that they have done the research and they render an opinion that the deal will work and if it doesn't work the law firm will be behind the client to support them in times of trouble. And typically when seeking "opinion letters" it is the norm to begin with the larger law firms, especially depending on how aggressive the strategy is. This law firm had only twenty professionals. So this told us that larger firms had likely passed on writing such an opinion letter.

West Capital also observed the technique on the part of Classic Star to make our clients feel "special" for being chosen for this strategy and this investment. Such an interpersonal strategy raises a lot of concerns for us in our practice. And so West Capital advised our clients that "this is not an appropriate strategy," "we cannot see how it works," and we advised clients to "avoid it." As it turned out two of our clients did avoid the strategy. But the third gentleman who was our client decided differently. He said that he understood what we were saying and that it might not work. But he said to us "my spouse really likes going to the Kentucky Derby" [Laughter]. This really was a true conversation. And he said that the deal "feels very important and very special. They made us feel at home and so we are going to do it." This client signed off on a waiver with regard to our advice. They went ahead and did the deal.

As it turned out, in the fall of 2007, in September, the IRS conducted a raid. Even if we assume for a moment that the strategy would have worked, the IRS found that Classic Star did not have enough horses for all of their clients. Even if the strategy would have worked, Classic Star was not able to satisfy necessary requirements. A long while after this, all of the horses were sold at auction, every client of Classic Star has been audited, one of the principals of Classic Star is still a federal fugitive on criminal charges, and about $800 million in tax penalties have been levied. And because the nature of the deal was such an outrageous stretch within tax law the client ended up having to pay all of the taxes that they owed as well as an extreme excise penalty on the tax So the medical doctor who chose to do it because he "felt at home" and his wife "liked the Kentucky Derby" was not able to apply the same sense of due diligence in his personal investments as he would apply to the surgeries he performed. In spite of red flags everywhere, prior to the deal, he chose to go ahead, and it ended up costing him a tremendous amount of money.

My second example involves a company called DBSI, which is a real estate management company. One of our West Capital clients has built a tremendous network that is many hundreds of millions of dollars in real estate. He has made a huge fortune in real estate. He has been in the real estate industry for more than thirty-five years and he understands his industry thoroughly. This client actually came to us after he had made the investment with DBSI. Our client had been introduced to DBSI because he had sold a property and DBSI offered him something called a 1031 exchange, which is a common practice in real estate as a tax shelter. The investment that DBSI offered was an eight per cent guaranteed rate of return. Our client told us that what had helped solidify in his own mind that this was a safe transaction for him was that the DBSI literature said, of itself, that it had over a hundred years of experience in the real estate world. And so our client felt very confident in investing with DBSI, or as we would learn, our client was overconfident. He presumed that because he had built years of wealth in real estate that the DBSI literature, with one hundred years of experience, was the key factor to confidence.

Unfortunately in May of 2008, DBSI declared bankruptcy. All of the guaranteed income that was to be there for our client is not there because it is in bankruptcy court. Also, because our client was so overconfident that he did not go through the due diligence that he otherwise would have executed, the structure of the investment was not good. Our client no longer owns the property, and the bankruptcy court does own it. Our client is now a general creditor, which means he has lost all his rights. And the hundred years of experience that our client assumed was like his own company, with thirty plus years of experience split among four partners, was nothing like that. The hundred years that DBSI advertised in literature was actually thirty-five realtors with an actual experience of two to three years experience each, which they advertised as one hundred years. And so my point with this example is that our client's overconfidence in his own business led him to make certain assumptions, without checking, when it came to making certain investment decisions with monies he had achieved from a sale.

These are two examples from experiences with clients of our firm, and we have others, when very smart people in their own businesses do not apply the same due diligence criteria when it comes to investing.

These otherwise smart people make assumptions with regard to investments with other agents. The assumptions are often driven strictly on an emotional basis, as it was in the first example. That individual was more concerned with his spouse being happy about the experience that the investment would supposedly bring than he was in understanding the deal itself. They do not think of the investment with the same critical process that they would in their own business. This is why firms like mine make sure that there is an independent custodian with our client investments. We do not run in house products or portfolios. We use independent and diverse managers so that no one single strategy can sink an entire portfolio. We spend time understanding clients like this and again, I emphasize their competence in their own business. But they need our help. In terms of financial investing they do need to have the advice of some professional who understands it, who is objective, and who really does go through all of the processes. Just because you are successful in a profession does not mean that the skill base will transfer to managing your portfolio. So with that in mind, thank you for listening to my examples.

Chris Cutler, CFA
Manager Analysis Services, LLC
New York, NY

Thank you Chris.

Chris Topolewski and I talked about what we would discuss before we arrived here today and I knew that the two examples he chose would be particularly amusing. But at the same time I just want to emphasize that what we are talking about are exceptions in the industry, and that the vast majority of what we look at are very solid investment managers, of high integrity, and with very good risk control. And I particularly want to emphasize that fact because I am about to discuss Madoff. Most of the alternative investment industry is not like that. Another footnote as I begin is that while Madoff is a huge scandal, there is another one going on right now called "Stanford," which has been in the press. Stanford was a bank based in Antigua, and I don't know who would want to put a CD in a bank in Antigua, but apparently eight billion dollars worth of investors did and in addition Stanford apparently advised on fifty billion dollars in total in wealth management. I don't have enough detail today to talk about that but I think that the Stanford story may be even more fascinating than Madoff in many ways. What Chris before me said, about the advisor not actually controlling the cash, is very important. In the case of Chris Topolewski's firm the client cash is held at Fidelity, State Street, or other independent institutions so that outside control is very important. In the new Stanford scandal, outside control did not exist and I will get in to why that is important, later on.

So I will now move into Madoff and, before I do I just want to comment on what I do. My own business is helping institutional investors conduct due diligence on their hedge fund managers. I started this business in 2003 and I don't have an exact number but I estimate that I've looked at 750 to 800 hedge funds in some capacity over that period of time. I know the industry well, I know what the issues are quite well. And over that period of time I was asked to look into one of the Madoff feeder firms and based on that experience I want to share my perspective with you. But first I would also comment that I think the media wants to tell their perspective on the story in their way. But when they do the media miss a lot of important complexities regarding what happened with Madoff. What Madoff was doing was very complex in many ways and because of the complexities there were/are some hugely intelligent people in the hedge fund investing community who are investors with Madoff.

You would think that a lot of what I do in due diligence is in regards to markets and analysis, and financial analysis, and risk management. And this is all true. But one of the things that I demand to do wherever possible is to meet the manager of the hedge fund. There is something about that personal interaction with a manager that provides cues or hints about the manager's personality or their stability. Sometimes I wish I had psychiatric training because hen I could get a lot more out of those personal meetings than I do now. But sometimes, with my limited intuition, it is possible to sense things that cause one to move away from a particular manager.

Now, going into Madoff: It is my opinion that there are often conceptual structures that exist that can perpetuate illusions. One of the key ones with regard to Madoff is that the existence of Federal regulation that insures business are real. And I think that people got a lot of comfort out of that with regard to Madoff. And another conceptual structure is that if there are strong independent credit ratings, and then people would be assured that an investment was pretty sound and safe. I think that this particular conception probably handicapped people when they were looking at subprime mortgages and other investments like that. The popular thinking seems to be that if the armies of financial analysts are reviewing the same issues, then that must insure that certain minimum considerations are met. If everyone else has looked at it, then what incremental value can you, as an independent analyst possibly add to any evaluation. The psychology of that kind of thinking has been out there for quite a while. And also a popular conception is that if there is a strong pedigree behind a manager, you don't need to be as careful as you otherwise would with regard to due diligence. In fact I have encountered that psychology in many cases. So given the brief outline of these conceptions I have provided a framework for discussing Madoff.

Some of the Madoff issues were blatant problems from a due diligence perspective. One of them has to do with some of the Madoff feeders. In looking at just one of the feeders it seemed that the sheer volume of trading that Madoff alleged to have done, both in options and in equities was too much to be credible. People believed that Madoff was running in the mid-twenty billions. And in that range, the amount of equity trading he was supposedly doing, even in the largest capitalization stocks should have been moving the market. But in fact if you added up all the trade tickets together and look at a particular day volume, the amount that he was trading was well under the illusion. But even with that being the case, going through the market and buying those securities would cause them to move a lot, and it would make it very difficult for him to have been making as much money as he said he was making. I emphasize this on the stock side because a lot of attention has been placed on the option side that supposedly would move the markets. So this was clearly a problem that an expert in the markets should have picked up on. But people believed that maybe Madoff was making money by front running the trade orders. This means that because he had a securities brokerage firm he would get orders from clients to trade stocks. Then somehow he would take that information and he would trade in front of it and that would make his trades more profitable. But this creates a clear conflict of interest between the two divisions of Madoff. He was supposed to be acting in the interests of the clients on the stock trading side but if he had been doing as I describe he would have been making money in the asset management side. This was a conflict of interest.

Another problem in my business is that when you conduct due diligence on a hedge fund manager, you want to insure that there is real talent in the shop. You look at the biographies of the traders involved and you talk to people who have left a particular firm to see what their perspectives on management might be. Maybe there were problems with the individuals, maybe with the strategy, and so on. But there has always been great difficulty finding any employee who ever left Madoff. So what this should reveal is that key talent other than just one person was missing in the Madoff firm. And a further huge problem was that Madoff himself actually controlled the money. You would send money to Madoff securities and you would trust that they were doing what they said they were doing with it. This is a big due diligence issue in hedge funds. But the same thing is also true with places like Merrill Lynch and some other brokerage dealers. You send them your money and you are trusting that they are doing what they say they will do.

Some other things were particularly problematic with Madoff. It is difficult to think about these things with hindsight. But Madoff provided 100 percent transparency to his feeder funds on what he said he was doing. At the end of every week he would send tickets to all of the feeder funds showing every single trade. And you could send an army of accountants to look at those trades and everything would check out against his claims of performance and against trades on the exchanges and you wouldn't find a problem. But what was very awkward about this was that the tickets that Madoff sent out were paper tickets. He was running as a premier broker-dealer, he should have had ample resources to the best technology ever, but he was sending paper tickets in the 21st century that technology had made obsolete a decade earlier. And a second issue was that none of the tickets were time-stamped so you wouldn't really know what time of day they were occurring so that you would have additional data to help verify whether the transactions were real.

The Madoff feeder-structure was very awkward because the distributors of Madoff were making disproportionate amounts of money relative to the services that marketers would earn in other roles of other hedge fund managers. From a legal perspective, though I am not a lawyer, when you are concerned about conflicts of interest inside of a hedge fund, one of the things you actually look for is whether there is other family members involved with the business. Part of the reason for this is that under United States law family members cannot be compelled to testify against each other. In addition, Madoff's auditor was an unknown, small auditor. Not only was he unknown, he was auditing the securities firm of Madoff. As far as anyone knows now, no external auditor was auditing all of the accounts that were actually running the money.

So in retrospect now, these problems I have discussed with Madoff appear to have been obvious. But even three years ago I was telling all of my clients that there were potential problems with Madoff. I did not suggest that he was running a Ponzi scheme. But I did think he was taking the money and doing something with it other than what he was telling the investors. But I had no further information other than my gut for the reasons discussed because I did not know anyone inside Madoff. There just seemed to be enough reasons not to put money there. Nevertheless most people did not accept my advice to stay away from Madoff when it was offered. I have some ideas as to why people did not take the advice to stay away but also I am interested in feedback from today's audience.

First of all, to accept the criticisms against Madoff required a leap of faith. Most people don't have the repertoire of abilities required to see problems in equity or options trading to detect potentially fraudulent problems. It is also hard for anyone but the most sophisticated in the business to understand hedge fund strategies well enough to determine what might be unrealistic or something that might get flagged by regulators. It takes an unusual repertoire of seasoned skills to raise the appropriate questions. Also the key leap of faith was simply to think, "How could something like this be happening?" How could someone be running twelve billion dollars, for twenty years, be regulated by the SEC and FINRA, had audits in the past, acceptable due diligence in the past and be potentially fraudulent? To think such a thing would have been to think that the entire financial infrastructure of the US economy had something wrong with it. People didn't think that the SEC and policy makers would ever let something so fraudulent ever happen. And many of my clients pointed out to me that Bernie Madoff himself was a former chairman of the NASDAQ. He ran a significant securities operation that accounted for over ten per cent of the daily volume in US equities. So people would say to me: "How can I accept your advice to stay away from this, Chris?" To my mind it was a huge conceptual problem that people couldn't handle. For some people who could overcome the conceptual problem in the first place, then the potentially fraudulent problems became obvious. But the issues involved are very complex and it is very hard to contradict what seems to be so solid.

In my work of due diligence I look at many hedge fund strategies. Some are very simple and others are quite complex. And my experience has been that in the middle of complexity we find self-doubt. Peoples limited cognitive ability to comprehend problems in such a way as to see "fraud" is not only very hard. It is also creating a substantial legal risk for oneself to suggest wrongdoing. In my opinion this was something that aided Madoff. I think that many people were afraid of being sued, thought that they had limited power up against someone like Madoff and so they maintain illusions within themselves. Just as there was an illusion of actual transparency with Madoff. I myself worked at a major broker dealer for eight years. I was a regulator at the Federal Reserve Bank of New York. I have had the rare privilege of being privy to many aspects of what is otherwise very complex analysis. It is clear to me that even a regulator is likely to miss many of the potential issues involved in wrongdoing.

Due diligence is the process of distilling an infinite set of information into a finite set of decision variables. That cannot be done perfectly. There will be compromises. Knowing where these will occur is difficult. The best due diligence analysts realize they are not perfect. The best thing that investors can do is to be risk aware instead of risk averse and try to manage what their risks are so that they can understand their exposures. Many of the weaknesses that were true of Madoff were true of other prominent, well renowned hedge fund managers that are first-in-class businesses. After the financial crisis scandal some are moving away from self-administration and hiring external administrators. This does not mean that the first-in-class firms had been doing wrong. Rather they like to control the quality of their product, which is understandable. With Madoff, the motives were different, as we have seen.

Those are my comments on Madoff. I am going to pass this on now to Elliot Noma and I welcome the Q & A that will follow.

Elliot Noma, PhD
Managing Director,
Garrett Asset Management
New York, NY

Thanks Chris. What I am going to try to do is that I am going to try to talk in terms of Madoff and other things that we see in the financial world right now. I guess I could probably summarize my short presentation, as "Money is the Meaning of Life." And I am going to start where Chris left off, in terms of the due diligence process. Part of the issue in terms of the due diligence process is it is a very human activity. Basically, when we are doing due diligence it is very much like going out on your first date, in some ways. You are trying to do an evaluation and you are hoping that the evaluation will be as positive as possible. In a way you are entering the process in the first place because you are willing to spend the time and effort with a confirmation bias, at the beginning.

So you start with that process in mind, and you have to think in terms of the other players who are also doing the same thing that you are doing, in terms of deciding whether to get into a particular investment or not. Steve Greenspan talked about the gullible investors, and I think that I will list myself in that category, even though I never invested directly in Madoff. But I am always trying to give the benefit of the doubt to what I am looking at. For example, I can look at a manager and say that the manager is not giving me transparency. This is not necessarily good on the surface of it but I can understand the argument saying "Well, this is a sensitive strategy and you are asking me as an investor to be brought inside the tent". Another thing is that there is a level of mystique about incomplete transparency and having a person's potential financial future, to an extent, in my hands. For example if the strategy is so good and so powerful, then there must be a real secret sauce. So for every positive in the evaluation, the due diligence process forces another way of viewing things.

The second thing I want to talk about Madoff is, as Chris mentioned in his remarks, the questions about the theories that people brought up in terms of how Madoff was making his money. There were analysts who looked at Madoff and said that he must be doing something else there. But if they followed that line of thinking they would/should has realized that he was running a money management firm and he was a large market maker. There must be something within Madoff where the two groups are talking to each other for competitive advantage. Yet as financial professionals we know that there is a wall between these parts and information should not flow between them. We all know better. But there was also the idea that the SEC has looked into the investment. This guy Madoff must be pretty sharp. So if the people in the best position to catch this management firm in a fraud has not done so then "I," a new investor, will be okay. In other words this is just the pure greed of the investor and a willingness to look the other way because the smart money management firm isn't getting caught.

The third thing is Bernie Madoff himself. I never had the opportunity to interview him or anybody in his firm, so I can't really say whether this is part of his dynamic. But he was a highly successful market maker. He had a long history, very prominent in the regulatory world with very high personal status. But then looking at the economics of his business, he's got a moneymaking business and a money management business. He has been around for more than two decades and during this time business rules have changed. Stocks used to trade at eighths; now they trade at a penny. Hence market makers and the level of competition among them were harder. The spread was smaller. So in order to keep up his successful franchise in the market making part of the business he had to think about where else he would make money. And another way to make money was in Madoff's own other half of the business. So this becomes more than just a question about fraud and cheating but what is going on in Bernie Madoff's head when he moves to this conflict of interests.

The bigger picture, as I had mentioned at the beginning with "Money as the Meaning of Life" causes me to think of the famous sociologist Max Weber. He was probably the most famous for talking about Protestantism being one of the foundation elements of capitalism and money and finance as misplaced religious quests in terms of looking for meaning. How does this manifest itself? I have already talked about possible manifestations with Madoff. But there are three other things to talk about in terms of money being a religious experience.

First of all who in the audience remembers the movie "Trading Places"? Good. I see hands on that. And you may remember that the basic premise of that movie is that you have two very rich people who decide to conduct a social experiment. They will take a successful person in their firm and reduce him to poverty and make it look like he is also a criminal and see what happens to him. Then they have another person who is a street-smart guy, with nothing else going for him, and they bring him to the firm to prove that he will be successful. It was an experiment in the movie. What is less well know is that in 1983 when the movie was made there was also a program that was taking place in Chicago. There were two well-known traders, Richard Dennis and Bill Eckhart who had a similar conversation. They asked: "Can we take people off the street and make them successful traders?" In other words can we give them the religion, or the secret sauce? And these guys brought in a class in '83,'84,'85. My point here is that because people believe that there was a "secret sauce" they were willing to try it, presume that they would/could learn it and be successful at it. In fact next Tuesday at the Marriott Times Square there is a similar kind of program happening called "Trader Tech" taking place. Anyone can go there and try. Registration is free.

The next thing I want to mention is Warren Buffett. He is obviously one of the great investors of the twenty-first century and his annual gathering of his investors is like a pilgrimage, like going to Mecca. He does presentations and things are twittered about what Buffett thinks. It becomes like received knowledge in terms of how it is utilized. So once again the basic point is that money is more than just money. It involves ego in terms of the due diligence, in terms of advisory work, and so on. Confirmation biases, rejections of recommendations, greed and envy are all things that fit together in many ways.

I want to end my comments with mentioning how much I enjoyed Mitchell Wilson's summary remarks this morning of your earlier papers. He talked in terms of greed and the movie *Wall Street* with Michael Douglas and Charlie Sheen. This was the movie of the famous "Greed is Good" speech by Michael Douglas' character, Gordon Gecko. But at the very end of the movie Charlie Sheen finally understands what Hal Holbrook, head of the trading desk, has been talking about in term of man staring in the abyss, in understanding the concept of life, and being in his penthouse apartment saying "Who am I?" Because, at that point, money has so consumed him that Charlie realized his whole being is tied up in being a successful rich person. Fortunately he is able to step back, and that is the moral of the film.

The other thing that Mitchell Wilson's review mentioned was the level of ferocity of greed. If any of you have read any of Donald Trump's books or parts of them, the ferocity shines through them. Trump is always looking for the deal. It sort of transcends the money in the process. This is him: who he is. And then, more recently, there is the controversy about bonuses. What has not been said so much in the press is that bonuses for many Wall Street people and traders go beyond basic need. It is really a question of keeping score. "Why did this person make $5-million and I only made $3-million—or whatever the number is?". And that is the point where you realize that you are talking about status in a society; you are talking about the creation of a demand. Wall Street has done a great deal as far as promoting the idea that if you are a god; you are going to get paid like a god. That is better than annual reviews, which are better than hosting charity events, or sponsoring conferences. It is the best thing on earth when you get paid. In other words, Wall Street has created the demand, so now you have to step up in this world, because that is what matters. And with that I will stop and look forward to the discussion.

AUDIENCE DISCUSSION

Leslie Shaw,
Moderator

My remarks are off-the-cuff here so please bear with me if the organization of ideas is not what it could be, given more time to reflect. Nevertheless as I listened to these presentations we could hear each of these gentlemen re-iterating their sense of disbelief in the inabilities of their clients, and often even their peer professionals to recognize significant indicators in information that should have led clients to reject an investment opportunity. Steve Greenspan showed courage and humility in sharing with us that even a psychologist who studies gullibility is potentially vulnerable.

Within the framework of the theme of this symposium we have focused on the psychoanalytic pathological or character-structure flaws that reflect archaic greed or other personal longing that is inherent in investment decisions. The client decision processes that our speakers described were anomalous to the otherwise significant rational decision-making processes that these clients had exhibited within their own professions. Both Chris T. and Chris C. shared their extreme frustrations with regard to clients who seemed to be chasing illusions. Our speakers had been hired to do due diligence. And yet all possible disconfirming evidence about their clients' investment opportunities under consideration were ignored in the pursuit of the fantasy; or so it seemed. So from a psychoanalytic point of view we see our professional speakers seeming to have to deal with what we might call the "split-off" aspects of their clients.

Psychoanalytically we would be able to suggest that the clients in question did not want the anxiety of the contradictory data that our two Chris's had presented to them. Our speakers tried to bring the contradiction to client conscious awareness, but to no avail. And yet are we really surprised? Clinical psychoanalysts in this audience deal with the individual struggle of ambivalence within their patients that is so often at the heart of the psyche. Within patient sessions you all see the certainty of a one-sided perspective that patients reveal in relation to their powerful objects. It takes considerable working through to arrive at a resolution of the inner tension that resolves the ambivalence. The much safer haven for the patient to be free of anxiety is often to remain certain of either an idealized perspective or a rejection of the object. In primitive pathologies that exhibit more extreme splits the behavioral breakdown, as we saw with

Jeff Stern's Elliott Spitzer, is at a de-coupled distance from the Elliott Spitzer who was the ruthless pursuer of the greed for power in others that he did not want to accept within himself. We are psychoanalysts and so we tend to see all of this in terms of our understanding of pathology.

But as much as our purpose here today is about psychoanalytic expression and questioning I would like to suggest to you that another behavioral discipline, that of behavioral decision making or behavioral economics, also has something to offer the observations about which we hear this morning. Eliot Noma touched on this field when he spoke about "framing" or the context within which information is presented to decision makers. Mitchell Wilson included it in his summary when he spoke of the (behavioral) economist Akerlof, a Nobel Laureate, who used the role of environment as a factor in human identity and its significance for enacting social policy. In Mitchell's view these behavioral economists have sometimes "stolen" concepts from psychoanalysis but given them a behavioral name while not giving psychoanalysis any credit. For example he pointed to the work of Erikson and Lacan that far preceded behavioral economist interest in identity.

Nevertheless having been trained as a Ph.D. in behavioral economics, before acquiring my own psychoanalytic training, I would like to say that the two psychological disciplines may have more to offer each other than not; that potentially they might become (even) more than friendly relations. I say this because one of the things that psychoanalysts have done poorly is to size their ideas in a way that is understandable and useful outside of the consulting room. And yet all of the stories told by our gentlemen above had to do with a phenomenon that behavioral economics has termed "overconfidence in judgment."For behavioral economists the term does not imply pathology. The phenomenon is ubiquitous and often measurable. As a brief exercise here this morning let me ask you to consider some of your own judgments, beliefs, and hypotheses: for example, you consider one of your own friends to be devious, or you might hold the hypothesis that the Democrats are responsible for inflation, etc. Although our own judgments and beliefs may be considered as hypotheses to be tested, we are generally quite confident in their truth without ever formally testing them. The behavioral decision and economics discipline has contributed considerable science that shows that the lack of search for disconfirming evidence within and among human beings is a ubiquitous phenomenon. Getting at our own due diligence must involve a willingness to attempt to falsify our own hypotheses, even if that hypothesis is blatantly unrealistic. Another twist on what I am getting at is this: A behavioral finance person would say to us here today that the task into which Chris Cutler was pouring his heart and soul, unfortunately must involve "a willingness by his clients to test those intuitive ideas, that so often carry the *feelings* of certitude within his clients. It is very much like the involvement and *readiness of* the patient to be able to *hear* the interpretation.

Unfortunate as it may be the scientific evidence is clear that people simply do not actively search for disconfirming evidence. And while they don't necessarily ignore outcome feedback people only selectively attend to certain aspects of it. By being more selective in attention to information the individual can have the self-experience of receiving more positive outcome feedback about his judgment ability even if the true correlation between the judgment, ex ante, and the outcome, ex post, is a low correlation. (Sort of like the correlation between yield on monetary investment and "my wife likes to go to Kentucky," per the Chris Topolewski story). Is this really so different from the patient who comes, for many sessions, and reports only the positive (or negative) perceptions of a good (or bad) object?

Much as it might be part of our own fantasy, we cannot say that the answer to the problems we have heard these two days is to psychoanalyze everyone. But what we do have to bring to the table is the emotional factor that is the missing link that gets at the human construction of meaning. What we might learn in the next decade, especially as neuroscience continues to validate the organic basis of the libidinal, in the terms of "seeking" aspects of Freud's theory, is that the Behavioral Decision and Economics people may be able to help psychoanalysts develop a technology, especially where large organizations need to process huge quantities of information while at the same time contain the human anxieties within the organization. Hopefully, if the two fields begin to talk to each other we might develop some measurement in time that will warn when human structures are beginning to overheat so that we can enact responsible interventions before breakdown occurs.

There is a worthwhile academic paper in the *American Journal of Psychiatry,* 1999, on the "Future of Psychoanalysis." The author is the Nobel Laureate in biology, Eric Kandel. The paper is beautifully and brilliantly written. The future that he hopes for us is an eventual integration with cognitive neuroscience.

Okay, given these brief highlights of the salient issues that seemed to be in common among all of our panelists, we want to get in some audience questions for everyone. This has been an intense morning of papers and panel after a very stimulating day yesterday. We are already running a little bit overtime so with that in mind lets go to questions.

Audience Member: My question is for Chris Cutler. Chris, as you were talking I was very curious if you would share your experience, your personal experience of, as you were describing, advising people against investing in the Madoff fund. Running up against the dissonance of responses from people. What did that feel like to you? Because in the context of what we are looking at now, there was almost a rush that the markets had been caught up in. You had the experience of being in it and yet you were standing apart with regard to advice that you were giving some of your clients. Can you tell us what it felt like to go home at the end of the day?

Chris Cutler: I don't understand the question, are you referring to December 12th, or are you referring to when I advised people not to be in Madoff?

Audience Member: I'm referring to when you were advising people that the Madoff fund really didn't add up in the time period when there was all sorts of evidence that was fairly believable to people who wouldn't have even been considered gullible and you are there saying, "Well, I wouldn't actually advise investing with Madoff", and they look at you like, "are you dumb or what?" What did that feel like? I want to know, personally, what does it feel like to say no in the midst of a mad rush?

Chris Cutler: Well, humorously I will object to the question because I was told that I wouldn't be psychoanalyzed when I was here. [Laughter].

Audience Member: No, this is not a psychoanalytic question, this is curious personal question.

Chris Cutler: It was extremely difficult. I have to tell you, from a business perspective, I lost potential clients by telling them that "you guys should not be in Madoff" when there were a lot of problems, because no matter how gently I put my concerns to people, they did not want to hear negatives regarding their investment decisions. Everybody in finance thinks they are smarter than everybody else. And while I mean that mostly with humor, people have pride in what they do. So when you tell them that they may be wrong it doesn't go over too well.

But I'm a veteran; I can take it. So I stand my ground. I work at having great integrity behind what I do. It was very frustrating, in answer to your question, because I tried extremely hard in a number of cases to convince them that they shouldn't be in Madoff. But I have been in similar situations before.

Audience Member: Thank you.

(Next) Audience Member: Even though I assiduously read everything on Madoff, I still don't understand the extent of the fraud that he perpetrated. *The Times* came out with a statement, I believe, that he had actually not made a trade—an actual trade—for twenty years, twenty-five years, something like that. I think you are saying that he actually sent false tickets out too. What other false things happened? What was the extent of the actual fraud?

Chris Cutler: One of the characteristics of this and other frauds is pulling in other legitimate organizations that add legitimacy to the fraud. There were roughly fifteen feeder funds with Madoff. I was not an expert at the feeder funds at the time of all of them but I certainly knew a couple of them. The funds were audited by auditing firms with names you would recognize. So if the auditing firms were looking at the funds, and the auditors supposedly have their own procedures to verify transactions as real, then there is legitimacy that becomes a part of the fraud. Also there was due diligence done on Madoff as an individual and that was clean; for example, firms that did background checks on him and police records and things like that. There were also prominent investors who understand hedge fund strategies. They looked at it and despite the criticisms that later came out in the press about trading strategies, the hedge fund experts had been ok with it. So it is a fraud that occurred at many, many levels.

Audience Member: So did he actually send false statements out every month?

Chris Cutler: Absolutely. I have seen the trade tickets. Roughly at the end of every week, he would stuff envelopes full of paper trade tickets of equities and options that he was alleged to have traded. And you can look at every one of those trades and look at the price of the securities traded that day and it would be in the range of what in fact had traded. If I recall correctly, the average trade was across thirty stocks, and then one or two equity options.

Audience Member: And to his clients he sent completely false information each month.

Chris Cutler: Every month, to all the feeders. And the transaction feeders were consistent apparently across all of the feeders.

Audience Member: That takes a lot of talent.

Chris Cutler: It takes in my opinion more than one person, let's put it that way. I believe that there were other statements that were sent out. I believe that all of the clients got monthly statements. I did not look at the retail side of it. But the retail clients also got statements. The entire scheme was elaborate and required systems and people to put the thing together, in my opinion.

(Next) Audience Member: I'd like to thank everyone for what I have been learning in each of the topics, yesterday and today. And I would like to start with the concepts of greed and gullibility. To me they sound like addictions. I think greed is an addiction just by itself. It doesn't matter what the greed is about because it is a repetition over and over and over. The other piece of it is that greed and gullibility are connected in that in each situation the individual is looking to be special, or have something special that other people don't have. And the greed is to satisfy unmet needs. The purpose is to have something special or to *BE* someone special. The other final thing is what you just talked about Dr. Shaw and that is the need for mourning. In the case presentation yesterday the patient was a really good example in that he had developed enough trust in the therapist that when he finally came to his crisis he was at a point where he could mourn and cry and only because of that could he move on. I believe that mourning is so misunderstood, whether it's the War in Iraq, or whatever crisis has occurred, before people can move on.

Stephen Greenspan: I would like to say one brief thing. And that is that Emile Durkheim in his book on anomie said that people are actually more likely to commit suicide when the business cycle is going up than when it is going down. Personally, I have grown from losing money and I know people who have lost a lot more than I have and who have grown from it. The one thing that they got out of it was that maybe their values needed to be re-calibrated so that they could be more satisfied with what they have, rather than constantly wanting to keep up with everyone else. So no one wishes this kind of thing to anyone but perhaps there are benefits to be had from the experience.

(Next) Audience Member: Question with regard to applied psychoanalysis: It has been touched upon here. So if we look at greed, oral, primitive greed, as something that deeply affects the world, our country, and the people in it, what kinds of questions does psychoanalysis need to ask? How can the things we know raise important questions outside of our offices? Because what we know doesn't get spread round too far beyond the walls of the different learning institutions and offices that we have. This is a big question to me. I don't know if it is a question that someone cares to address at this point.

Leslie Shaw: When you say what kinds of questions should we be asking, I have a perspective. I have spent a lot of years working in the real world and not as a clinician. But the richness of the psychoanalytic literature and all that it has done in such a wonderful way in terms of clinical work is fantastic. I find myself remaining stunned that given the many fine psychoanalytic scholars, and we have heard some of them at this conference, that there was a time when nonmedical people were not going to be accepted for psychoanalytic training. One of our speakers at this conference presented a paper on the class action lawsuit that was necessary to allow non-medical people to be trained in psychoanalysis. So I just wonder if there is something about the history of the profession, and I think that Freud himself thought that if psychoanalysis was left in the hands of the medical profession he feared for psychoanalysis and he himself really hoped that it would be taken to an applied level. I find myself a little bit stunned that there isn't more of a public relating of what psychoanalysis knows to the public phenomena that we see. I think that we need to do more of disseminating of our own questions in a more public way. That certainly does not mean giving information about the patient. But the thinking from Freud to Winnicott to Kohut and so on and so forth should be conveyed in more publicly usable ways. Perhaps we need to think about how to size psychoanalytic ideas for a broader marketplace. Something that astounded me when I was doing PhD work, and then subsequently a psychoanalytic candidate, was how much the time series of psychoanalytic theory and what we know about from where Freud started, to the later British School, how much of that literature in a way paralleled what the history of economic thinking was writing about. So I think that the psychoanalytic profession has been remiss in not looking for parallels. And I apologize for such a long-winded answer but you got me started.

(Next) Audience Member: I very much enjoyed all of the presentations yesterday and today and I have learned a lot. It integrates with my having treated a few very wealthy people and what I see. I think that maybe the fact that they come for treatment means that they are healthier than a lot of people. But I have seen a lot of early childhood issues and their difficulty in resolving them. In some cases, they thought that making money would resolve them. Well, they made plenty of money but they still struggle, in many cases, with the same conflicts that they had when they were half the age that they came to see me. I wonder how can people learn about this if they don't have a chance to have the situation of a patient. What are the parallels in other issues? There is a lot of psychopathology that people don't have control over unless they come to see somebody.

Leslie Shaw: We are not going to be able to psychoanalyze everybody and we go way amuck if we try or say that everybody should. Let us just try to take a step back in a simple way. If we can communicate more the understanding, such as what we are hearing at this conference, it is that people are dealing with what is going on in their own inner world and what is going on in that world is dealing a little bit with what is going on in the inner world of a dysfunctional organization. I cannot specifically answer your question. I don't think we can end up with everybody being psychoanalyzed. But clinging only to trying to get people into treatment isn't what I think is going to get us over the hump. I will commend to you that there is a fellow who is doing a very good job of it and you can download it. His name is Manfred Kets DeVries who is at the Insead Business School in France. Kets DeVries is doing wonderful work in executive training programs. They have recently put a podcast, at least audio, on the web. He talks about wanting to show these people how we can connect to great thinkers and again, this is the way he says it, he "wants to pull together John Maynard Keynes and Sigmund Freud". He wants to pull together economic thinking with somebody it has never been put with before, namely Freud. And Kets DeVries point is that everybody shouldn't be psychoanalyzed. But if we can begin to nudge people in a way that they think in terms of an inner world that drives some of their experiences, and that this takes place in an organizational inner world that may be dysfunctional, then in his opinion we begin to make progress. Psychoanalysis has remained isolated for too long. We haven't communicated with other social sciences especially, and I think that is to our detriment.

(Next) Audience Member: Actually I have one question, one hypothesis, and one comment. [Laughs} First the question: I was speaking to a friend the other day that invests in a hedge fund. She said to me: "I don't trust this guy but I think he can make me money". So she invested anyway. So I am wondering with all these red flags flying around Madoff, whether one of the motives in people investing in his fund was awareness, on some level, that this guy might not be kosher. That he might be doing something not right but the SEC has not caught him, and I want to be part of the deal. So I was wondering if anyone on the panel had encountered that or sensed it in any of your clients? That is the question. The comment was that there was a wonderful paper yesterday, which you did not hear, about gambling. And the idea was that in the moment between placing the bet and the actual outcome, there is a kind of suspension of time and a suspension of the limitations of human existence with a kind of denial of mortality and death; a real kind of moment of transcendence. My hypothesis is that that sense also applies to what goes on in these traders' desks and these hedge funds. They might not acknowledge that they are gambling, but I have a sense that the same psychology might be going on in their minds at the same time.

Elliot Noma: I can speak as a portfolio manager that clearly you do have the sense, re trader experience, that generally what you do is that you will trade a portfolio which is called a paper portfolio, which means that you are simulating the trades. This is how portfolio managers train. If successful at simulated trades you will then go into real trading but there is a marked difference in terms of experience. And it is not a question of money; it is a question of the level of commitment that takes place. And a lot is at the point when you are saying this is what I want to buy or sell. So there is a big difference there and this means a totally different feeling in terms of time, in terms of framing the experience. This goes back to the Behavioral Decision psychologists Kahneman and Tversky in terms of framing. People do things differently and experience differently as a result of the change in frame.

CLOSING

Arnold D. Richards: The hour is late and I think I would like to conclude because I am supposed to have the final word. First of all, the world has changed, and what goes on in the world has an impact on our own practices. I think there has been, for decades, a tendency for us to think that the world is the consulting room and that what happens "out there" doesn't matter. Analysts were being faulted when they looked at reality and were told: "It is only the fantasy that counts." People talked about this before the Nazis in Vienna, when the world was coming apart. Should the analyst be concerned with what is going on? And to what extent? Some analysts took the pure position that they were not concerned.

But this can no longer be the case. Inevitable questions arise: How much do we as analysts need to know about finance, our patients financial situation, and the decisions they make? To what extent is it our job to help our patients decide what to do? Are there two worlds—the analytic world and the real world? Is this compartmentalized in terms of a totally separate part of the world? These are not questions that have easy answers. When your patient invests with Madoff, and announces, "I cannot see you anymore" or, "I cannot see you anymore because my parents invested in Madoff," the hypothetical becomes the real.

What we have been involved in at this conference is really a first. We are participating in a very unique kind of dialogue and exchange. The interchange we have had here between analysts and financial gurus is rare at an analytic meeting. We need more of this kind of interaction if we are to survive as practitioners and psychoanalysts. Our organizations may not be able to survive when their portfolios are impacted by events in the real world.

I want to thank all of the panelists who participated in the conference and the audience that listened and responded. It has been a terrific meeting. Thank you all for coming.

REFERENCES

GREENSPAN, S. (2008). *Annals of Gullibility: Why We Get Duped and How to Avoid It.* Westport, CT: Praeger.

KANDEL, E.R. (1999). Biology and the Future of Psychoanalysis: A New Intellectual Framework for Psychiatry Revisited. *American Journal of Psychiatry* 156:505–524.

NEW HOPE FOR SCIATICA

End Your Pain Now with Solutions Even Your Doctor Won't Tell You About

DUNCAN McCOLLUM D.C.

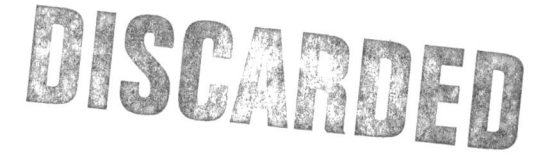

ISBN: 978-19-5-036797-9

Published by

LIFESTYLE ENTREPRENEURS PRESS

If you are interested in publishing through Lifestyle Entrepreneurs Press, write to: *Publishing@LifestyleEntrepreneursPress.com*

Publications or foreign rights acquisition of our catalog books.Learn More: *www.LifestyleEntrepreneursPress.com*

Printed in the USA

Contents

A Note from the Author

As I sit in the process of writing this book, perhaps the biggest wake-up call in modern history has plagued our planet. Even as I sit and write these words, citizens of our country and in fact the whole world are quarantined or confined to their own homes. Entire cities and even countries have been shut down and all non-essential businesses have been asked to temporarily close their doors.

The “deadly” corona virus has arrived and with it came mass hysteria. The powers that be; government, nations, our own CDC and FDA let alone the World Health Organization has been turned on its ear.

This corona virus invisible to the naked eye has proven the biggest terrorist of all. It is almost like our planet has been invaded from outer space and we are defenseless to the aliens attack.

People are scrambling for supplies, things as common as toilet paper and paper towels are nowhere to be found. Shopping cart have been commandeered and slammed together as frantic citizens are vying for position grabbing boatloads of supplies off the shelves of local grocery store often leaving none and showing no regard for their neighbor.

Not since the last World War has the world realized such a threat to survival.

And yet perhaps out of the rubble and ruin of an inept and now defenseless health care system will rise a new awareness in the minds of the peoples of earth. For far too many years we have depended on Big Phama to "save-the-day" with the next new "miracle pill". Yet with the invasion of corona we are left defenseless. Or are we?

Did you know that the wisest and most powerful physician who ever walk this planet lives right inside of you? It reminds me of the 1939 movie called "The Wizard of Oz". For the entirety of the movie Dorothy was searching for a way home. She evaded, wicked

witches, flying monkeys and fell victim to patches of wild intoxicating poppies when the whole time she had the power to find her own way home. As Glinda the good witch of the North would finally reveal, all she had to do was click the heels of her ruby slippers together and repeat, "there's no place like home, there's no place like home". Inside every one of us dwells an incredible innate intelligence. It has a purpose and that purpose is to survive. And for eons this innate intelligence has ensured that we survive. It wasn't until the advent of the massive pharmaceutical cartel who put profit above the people, that we started down this path of "magic Pill" dependence. Don't get me wrong, I realize how much modern medicine has added to our survival and our overcoming of hitherto overwhelming epidemics, but perhaps with this paradigm shift, it is time for the individual to take back the control of his or hers own health.

And through the pages of this book, as we discuss new and innovative ways for us to heal our own body and in this volume specifically addressing the multi-therapeutic approach to sciatica, it is my goal and desire to help you not only address your sciatica, but to rise above the dependency of another for

your amazing health potential and take the reins and learn to guide your life to where you can flourish and prosper while enjoying excellent health.

With love,
Duncan McCollum

CHAPTER 1:

There Comes a New Dawn – Why Can't I Get My Pain to Go Away?

Dear Friend,

If you are reading this book, then you have already spent many hours, weeks, months, or years struggling with the unrelenting pain of sciatica. Perhaps you have had bouts of it, or even lower back pain with a hint of leg pain, numbness, or weakness. The scary thing is that maybe you feel that it is getting worse. It's likely that you've been flat on your back and in so much pain, but nothing helped, and you've wondered about the best way to end it all. I've been there myself, and I do understand.

Whatever the reason for your interest, I hope you find the answers you are looking for. If you are at

a point where you know that in order to heal your body so you can enjoy your life again, you need to change something. Then this book is ready for you.

Maybe you've discovered that all the different pain meds, injections, nerve burnings, physical therapies, and even surgeries that might have worked for others has failed to work for you. I understand how it could be hard to imagine that the content on the pages in this book could be of help to you. Please be encouraged because after thirty years in practice and having suffered from breaking my own back over fifty years ago, I have personally tried everything short of surgery. As a result, I became a pretty good judge of what can and can't be done to help. Don't give up.

There is one limiting factor here that is up to you – you have to not just want the pain to go away, but you must demand that it go away. If you are ready for this, then read on! There is hope, and by getting through the pages of this book, I know you can be helped!

In this book, you will discover exactly what you need to do to handle your pain, but also to actually understand that in order to truly get well, you will

have to eliminate the multitude of issues culminating in your health condition.

I understand that right now you just want relief. Having suffered for too many years myself, I know what it is like to live a life of quiet desperation, hoping and praying that the pain goes away.

You are about to find answers to questions like:

- Where did my symptoms come from?
- Why haven't I been able to be helped?
- Will I ever be able to end the pain?
- How long will my doctor keep me on pain management?
- Am I becoming addicted to pain meds and other drugs?
- Am I damaging my organs by taking these drugs?
- Will I ever get well?
- Do I need surgery?
- What about my future?
- Will I ever enjoy my life again?
- What, if anything, can be done about it?

Be encouraged; there is new hope on the horizon. Your pain relief just got a new friend and your future looks bright. There are new technologies out there

little known by traditional medicine and even by the alternative healthcare community. By getting an understanding of what is wrong and getting a grip on what things are causing your chronic pain and inflammation, you will be empowered to take your life back. Right now, it is important for you to make this decision, and that decision is, "If it's to be, it's up to me!" It's time to make a stand. If you do, there is hope and you can be helped!

CHAPTER 2:

How Do I Know? My Journey to Be Me!

My first inkling that something was wrong came about in first grade. We were learning how to make letters on that big, lined paper. I had a yellow crayon in my hand and had just crafted a perfect letter "C" when Miss Dworkin looked at my work and immediately proclaimed that I did it wrong; it was backwards. I was confused and remained so for several years. Rather than explain to me that a "C" pointed the other way, I was quickly labeled *dyslexic* and thrown down a long, dark, and humiliating path.

Things got worse in third grade when we were in circle time reading *See Spot Run* out loud to each

other. A boy named John, who was completely blind, sat next to me. John had just finished reading a beautiful passage about Spot, with only his fingers, mind you, and it was my turn. However, I could not read a thing on the page. I remember the sinking feeling inside of me as the rest of the class looked on with so many different expressions. That experience stayed with me, haunting me in my unconsciousness for decades.

Shortly thereafter, my family moved to Piedmont, a small town about twenty minutes away from Berkeley, California, so I was away from the constant re-stimulation brought on by that moment in Emerson Elementary. As anyone who's family relocated can tell you, this was a trying time to get through by itself, and I'll talk more on that later.

The next wakeup call happened at age twelve. It was a rainy, Saturday morning, and I was visiting my two best friends from the Berkeley. Billy and Andy were twins, but Andy was born twenty minutes earlier. For some reason, they were known as Billy and Andy, and that was what we always called them – Billy and Andy. Anyway, we were up on "Tight Wad Hill" above the Cal Berkeley football stadium trying to watch the Cal-Stanford game.

This is a huge rivalry in the Bay Area and known as "The Big Game;" it was not to be missed. As it was obvious the rain was not going to let up, Billy and Andy produced what was called a "tube tent" from somewhere. This was a cylindrical plastic tube you would take backpacking back in the day. You'd run a rope through it tying each end to a tree creating a shelter from the weather. Boy backpack equipment has come a long way. The cylinder shape of the tube tent only had two openings, and since Billy and Andy held those positions and would not share, I'd decided to climb up a tree to get a better vantage point. As fate would have it, I apparently used very bad judgment in choosing the branch for my perch.

When Cal got a touchdown against an opposing team, it was tradition that a cannon located close by on Tight Wad Hill would go *BOOM* proclaiming the score. My excitement for the score and my kneejerk reaction to the sudden explosion created enough force to overcome the tensile strength of my perch. Suddenly, the branch I sat on snapped, propelling twenty-five feet down to the steeply sloped, rain-soaked hillside. I landed in a seated position, and then slid several feet down the muddy

slope. I remember not being able to move or get a decent breath of air. Not only was the wind knocked out of me, but if I tried to move, searing pain shot through my body. It took a moment for Billy and Andy to understand the extent of my injury and that it was bad enough that it would require them to exit the warm, dry, comfort of their tube tent to render first aid. It also meant they were likely to miss the results of the Big Game. Finally realizing that I really could not walk on my own, they carried me, one on each side, the three-quarters of a mile home to my house.

My parents who were happily engaging in one of their traditional Big Game cocktail parties had already imbibed their martinis and crumpets, so they paid little attention to just another injury their "accident prone" son came home with. I think I was given Aspirin and shooed off to the TV room. In those days, little kids were to be seen but not heard. In the crowd of guests at the house that day were at least a handful of medical doctors, all friends of the family and most of them neighbors. Eventually mom did take me to the doctor, one of her friends. The doctor's conclusion was that I had sprained my back, which would heal in a few weeks.

As a young kid, your only real role models are your parents. If they do not pay attention to your pain other than feed you dope, you simply begin to think that your condition is normal; pain becomes a part of your life. Trying to do things like be comfortable on the couch watching TV or even trying to sleep was hampered by varying degrees of toothachy lower back pain. Even though the pain level would vary, it was always there.

I remember the first couple weeks in seventh grade, all the guys were trying out for football and Coach Mentor had us flat on our backs on the field doing the old style sit ups. This caused excruciating pain for me. I recall the unapproving look in his eye as he watched me struggle. It was like he thought I was being lazy or like he decided right then and there I was not one of his chosen. I felt like an outcast, as though he had just stopped seeing me. There were days it wasn't so bad; I could run and play tree-tag, flying through the branches of a large oak at the top of the Piedmont Park. But in the evening, I would pay the price, often with searing back and leg pain coupled with degrees of depression. This, of course, would lead to my continued consumption of various illicit substances purchased

in the darkened sanctions of the Piedmont Park as an attempt to cover up both the physical and mental pain associated with my broken body.

Today, I have so much compassion for children and am constantly blown away by parents who say, "he is so young, how can he possibly have back pain?" Oh, believe me, he can!

For the next several years, my complaints fell on callused ears with fingers pointing to a bottle of aspirin or some other form of painkiller. All the drugs did was mask the pain at best; the pain never went away.

In 1969, I just turned fourteen, living in the Berkeley Bay Area. Telegraph Avenue, which borders the Berkeley Cal Campus, was in turmoil. The Berkeley Riots in protest of the Vietnam War was in full swing. Then, on May 15th of that year, a day remembered as "Bloody Thursday," Governor Ronald Reagan unleashed California's National Guard on the demonstrators and all hell broke loose. As the Guard shot into the crowd, a student was killed and another blinded. Finally, Cal's Berkeley student body was accompanied by thousands of other sympathizers numbered over 30,000 from around the country in a town which was scarcely over 100,000

at the time. A line was drawn, and you were either on the side of the "Left" or the "Flower Children" (protesters) or the side of the "Right," conservative, war mongers. Needless to say, I fell to the Left. With this move started my fourteen-year experience with every kind of mind altering and body numbing drug imaginable. Frankly, I was lucky to survive.

"Turn on, tune in, drop out" became the battle cry of the new counterculture-era. This was a phase popularized by the psychologist Timothy Leary as he spoke in front of 30,000 hippies in San Francisco's Golden Gate Park. I didn't necessarily find a drug that would relieve my pain, but I was definitely distracted from reality, which in itself was welcome at the time. I started taking drugs that could be procured on the streets near Telegraph Avenue. As early as 1968, I began paying attention to the words of Grace Slick as she sang the Jefferson Airplane's song "White Rabbit;" you can fill in the blanks. And so for the next fourteen years, I followed the suggestions in the lyrics of that song and began my quest to replace the essentially ineffective pills my mom provided me and to lose myself in the psychedelic euphoria promises of an emerging generation.

At age twenty, I was the proud owner of a 1959 Dodge half-ton pickup that I had purchased from my friend Andy a couple years earlier. This made me everybody's friend. One day, two friends approached me, offering to buy the beer if they could use my truck to move a piano they were given. I couldn't turn down the free beer, so I agreed to help them move the piano. So, we drank the case of Busch Bavarian talls and then headed off to get the piano; that's the way you did it in those days. Since I was the biggest and had no idea that it wasn't normal to live in constant lower back pain, I took the back end of the upright grand while my two buddies took the front. As we worked to get the piano out of the garage, the two guys in front said, "Okay, we're clear, pick it up," so I lifted my end of the piano, only to hit the top of the garage door. I was in a stooped, precarious position when it hit, and my back gave out and I collapsed to the floor. I re-injured my back, badly.

This left me flat on my back on the living room floor of my house in excruciating pain. I laid there for three weeks – nothing helped, and I mean nothing. I had access to almost any and all drugs on the market, both legal and illegal, but nothing touched the pain.

As I lay there on the floor, my friend, Joani, gave me massages and fixed me meals. I don't think I ate much, and as much as I liked Joani, the massages didn't help. The bigger problem was that I hadn't had a bowel movement in a week, and I was beginning to get scared.

The pain in my lower back was a fifteen out of ten and the burning pain down my legs was intolerable. It was about this time that I truly considered ending my life. I was hopelessly handicapped at twenty-years-old. I had been in pain for eight years, and nobody seemed to believe me or really care. I was considering my options when two friends walked in and decisively told me they were taking me to a chiropractor they knew.

"A *what*?" I thought. I had grown up in the medical doctor community of Berkeley in the sixties. Chiropractic at that time was a four-letter work, spelled incorrectly at that – *kwak*!

As I tried to protest, these two friends picked up this ugly, motheaten, green couch that I hauled down from my dad's house in the bay area, and they put it in the back of my pickup. Then, against my will, they picked me up; I remember screaming from the motion. They put me on my couch in the back

of my own pickup and started driving me away to my destiny.

The next thing I knew, my friends carried me into some office where this beautiful midwestern goddess handed me some paperwork to fill out. If it weren't for her angelic, lily white complexion and her Snow White mannerisms, I would have tried to crawl away, scratching my way out with my fingers, which were the only things that worked at the time.

Soon, I was carried into Dr. York's back office. Wow, what a scary moment. He was dressed in polyester pants and wore a white patent leather belt and similar shoes. His shirt was unbuttoned one too many buttons and his short-cropped hair was scary. As I explained the piano incident to him, he nodded and took notes. After poking around on my back, Dr. York told me he needed x-rays of me standing. This was a problem because I hadn't been able to stand for three weeks. With some convincing from Dr. York, my friends held me up as this "doctor" took x-rays of my back. Then, Dr. York disappeared behind a door labeled "dark room." I had no idea what that meant, but I remember the strange noises coming out of there and couldn't help thinking of Dr. Jekyll and Mr. Hyde. It was that strange.

After what seemed like an hour in the "dark room," the doctor walked out and put an x-ray up on a light box. He pointed to a spot on the x-ray and said the magic words that changed my life, "When did you break your back?" He was the first doctor in all those years to take my pain seriously. I burst into tears. No one had diagnosed the crushed vertebra in all those years. All they offered were lousy drugs that didn't even touch the pain. Now it became very clear to me that the deleterious effects of all the drugs I had consumed would never fix the problem and would only cover up the symptoms. As time went on, I began to realize the drugs' effects in regard to my inability to read, thus furthering my dyslexia diagnosis from the first grade.

What he said next scared the hell out of me, but as a result, it changed my life forever. Now, remember, I could not stand up at all and was suffering from terrible lower back pain that also shot down my right leg. I hadn't had a bowel movement in a week, and I was seriously considering a dark and permanent alternative; I did not want to live life like that. But then Dr. York said five words that gave me a glimmer of hope, "I think I can help."

He went on to explain that the old fractured vertebra was basically pancaked so many years ago; it was squashed. However, because I was so young at the time of the injury, the bone was still "green," so when it broke, it squished, kind of like silly putty. He said that if that had happened to a grown-up, mature bone, it would have snapped into fragments. He said I was lucky I was young when the accident occurred. Yikes!

Next, Dr. York talked about my bowel function and that the new injury caused the bones and soft tissue to squeeze up against my spinal cord. He said that this was likely pressing not only on the nerves and causing pain, but also on the nerves controlling my bowels. He said he would be willing to try to give me a chiropractic adjustment to move the bone off of the nerve, but only under the promise that I would immediately go to the emergency room if it didn't work. The Golden Gate Bridge option sounded better as he went along. However, Dr. York did have me sign a paper to the effect that I would go the hospital if the adjustment failed to help. My friends were held responsible to drive me there as well. I was scared to death, so I agreed to his terms.

Next thing I knew, Dr. York placed me on his "adjusting table" in a sideways position and before I knew what happened he "jumped on my back." There was a loud snap, a jolt of pain down my legs, and I felt like I was about to black out. I hated doctors at this point and had no regard for that guy – I'd had it! The rush of adrenaline had me jump to my feet, and I was about to hit or lambaste him. Suddenly, I realized I was standing on my own two feet for the first time in three weeks. I was stunned, dumbfounded, and ecstatic all at once. I was still in pain, but it paled in comparison to the pain I'd been carried in with. I began to cry.

As Dr. York explained what just occurred, I felt hope for the first time in years. He described the term something like this: when some kind of physical, chemical, or mental force is exerted on the body, the resulting trauma can have minor or major effects. Often times the trauma is such that one or more spinal vertebra will slip out of place or get misaligned. He called it a "subluxation". He stated that usually within a few days the body will recover, the spinal segments will regain 100 percent of its expected motion, and the communication centers of the body will be intact, and all will be well.

He explained that occasionally, the body cannot right itself from the trauma and the vertebra does not regain proper motion or function. At this point, the spinal segment will start to breakdown, kind of like a tiny cavity in your tooth beginning to form. And just like a cavity, this subluxation can go undetected, that is until that moment it hits a nerve. I've had plenty of tooth aches to understand that concept only too well. So when he explained how a misaligned vertebra can compress the delicate spinal nerve causing any kind of disruption of communication to and from the brain, I got it.

I realized that I had experienced all three types of trauma in my life:

1. **Physical**: falling out of the tree and crushing my fifth lumbar vertebra
2. **Chemical**: all the drugs and alcohol I consumed to try to rid myself of the pain
3. **Mental**: the anguish associated with wondering if I would ever get well as well as any other tricks my mind played on me

If all these things combined were responsible for my ill health, then I could see a path to hope. I was interested.

Over the next few weeks and into the next several years, Dr. York continued to talk to me about chiropractic and this concept of the subluxation.

The Subluxation

Dr. York explained that there were only thirty-one pairs of spinal nerves exiting the human spine, and those thirty-one pairs of spinal nerve divide and divide until there is a branch communicating with all seventy-five trillion cells in the body. He explained how in 1895 a magnetic healer named D.D. Palmer discovered chiropractic. As the story goes, there was a janitor named Harvey Lillard working in D.D.'s office who had a hearing problem; in fact, he was practically deaf. One day D.D. asked permission to examine Harvey. What D.D. discovered was a large lump protruding on one side of Harvey's neck. D.D. determined that this must be a misaligned vertebra caused by an earlier trauma Harvey sustained. D.D. asked permission to try to correct the misalignment, and Harvey was game. So D.D., having a good understanding of spinal structure,

positioned Harvey's body in such a way that when he exerted a measured amount of impulse on the misaligned vertebra, there was a loud pop and the bone returned to its normal expected position. With that Harvey got off the table and proclaimed that his hearing had returned. And Chiropractic was born. As the story goes, D.D.'s son, B.J. Palmer, who was 14, happened to be in the office at the time and was enthralled with what he saw. B.J. Palmer eventually took over the chiropractic reins and became the developer of chiropractic. He postulated that "the power that made the body could heal the body," and spent the next many decades dedicated to the development of what is today the largest non-medical, alternative health care profession in the world.

Through B.J.'s ensuing research he developed a working definition of subluxation. Basically it goes like this: when two vertebra are misaligned, from whatever cause, and your body's innate intelligence is unable to correct it, the segments will wear incorrectly causing disc decay and spinal arthritis at that level of the spine. The pressure of the misalignment disrupts communication to and from the brain, causing dysfunction, and if unchecked, a disease process will develop.

I was fascinated with everything Dr. York talked to me about and made the decision, at that moment, that I wanted to do what he did; I wanted to become a chiropractor. The only problem was that I couldn't read, so the odds were not in my favor. It took me several more drug-addicted years to finally pull out of it.

One night, when I was around twenty-five years old, it was around "three o'clock in the morning" as the BB King song goes, I found myself about to have a heart attack. I had consumed so much alcohol coupled with opium laced weed, copious amounts of cocaine, methamphetamine, and any downers I could find that I almost overdosed. I remember standing in my music room frozen in place, scared, literally unable to move. My heart felt like it was about to burst out of my chest. I stumbled my way to the cliff above the ocean near my house and reflected, "If I don't quit these drugs and alcohol I will die." That was it; I quit on the spot. It was that moment during which my life changed; I had to get that low.

The path before me was not an easy one. But after several failed attempts at school, reversion to pain killing drugs, bouts of depression and

self-abasement, and not even being able to read a comic strip, thirteen years after Dr. York had administered that first chiropractic adjustment, I made it. It might have taken thirteen years, but with the help of Dr. York, my father, sister, and a few fellow students pulling me along, I was able to overcome my learning disability, my drug and alcohol addictions, and physical limitations, and make my dream came true. On September 22nd, five days after the 1989 Loma Prieta earthquake, I graduated as Dr. Duncan McCollum Doctor of Chiropractic, and Dr. Anthony York and his beautiful wife, Patricia, were there to wish me well. Against all odds and all obstacles, I made it.

Today, my life is amazing. I am dedicated to staying on the upper end of the learning curve. I have connected with some of the top doctors on the planet, and my days are filled with studying and learning the newest and latest science in health and regenerative medicine. I am so fortunate to have connected with heroes such as Dr. Dan Pompa who is considered the world leader in cellular healing and true cellular detoxification. He has engaged me as one of the elite doctors in the Health Centers of the Future, and the regenerative medicine movement. The HCF

docs are about forty-five men and women dedicated to constant study of the latest research and then implementing that, which has proven effective in our search to forward regenerative medicine. The learning curve is steep, and as my great friend and colleague Dr. Mindy Pelz says, "being connected to Dr. Dan Pompa is like constantly being hit in the face with the powerful blast from a fire hose. Just when you think you got it and have caught up, a whole new volume of scientific data hits you in the face." It's never ending, but it's the ride of a lifetime. I feel so fortunate to be included in his journey. He definitely keeps my head spinning. Recently, Dr. Pompa introduced me to a guy named Bill (that's all I know), and I am now part of a clandestine Russian-based study on "turning back the biological clock," I'd love to tell you about it, but I'd have to...well, you know how the story goes.

As a result of recent testing, I have discovered that my biological age is forty-two years old; although, my actual chronological age is sixty-four. This is according to the length of something called "telomeres." Telomeres, if you don't know, are little filaments extending out at either end of your DNA. Each time your cells divide, meaning your DNA

duplicates to create two cells from one, the telomeres get a bit shorter. Once the telomeres reach a certain length, the cell becomes useless and usually dies. However, often times these old cells don't die and wreak havoc on neighboring cells and your health in general. These old, senile or "senescent" cells can also mutate into cancer and other bad things.

As you make your way through this book and learn the new sciences and technologies that will allow you to get results never before attained in reducing sciatica, you will also learn more about things like telomeres and how new science is paving the way to reverse your biological age, reduce your chance of developing "age related disease," and help you live well into your twilight years, enjoying good health with a memory that works.

I know the first thing, and really the only thing, you are probably interested in right now, is the answer to the question, "Can you make my pain go away?" I totally understand, please sit tight as I break down the process in the next chapter.

CHAPTER 3:

The Three Sides to Healing

By this time, I'm sure that you have tried any number of treatments to help your pain. Maybe you've had some success – I hope you have. But what I want to establish here is the myriad of factors you should look at in order to get well.

If you are familiar with the health triangle, you know that each side stands for a separate aspect of health: physical, chemical, and emotional. When searching for the causes of any health condition, a thorough study of all three sides of this health pyramid is imperative.

Physical

Let's start with the most obvious part: the physical aspect. In your case, this is what your spinal column consists of and how it works. Hang in there with me. This is an important starting point. There is an old adage that goes, "You can't be the adverse effect of that which you understand." What I mean by this and how it relates here, is that the better you understand how your body communicates with itself and how it goes about healing via its innate ability, the more you will be able to assist it in furthering its healing abilities. To this point, I remember when I first stepped into the anatomy lab, first quarter of chiropractic college. I took anatomy at Cabrillo College in Aptos and had a pretty good understanding of the body. Being dyslexic, I couldn't read, but through touching, feeling, observing, and exploring, there was no stopping my depth of understanding. I mean this to say this was in my learning wheelhouse.

What struck me then, and even today, while dissecting our human "volunteer," is that when I got to the nerves, as they exited the spinal column, they were actual physical things. From all the explanations I received growing up from would be spinal

experts, I understood the nervous system to be just some current that somehow flowed through the body. I was blown away by the hard, cordlike nerves, which exited the spinal column and then divided again and again until they reached every single one of the seventy-five trillion cells, which make up the body. This knowledge alone went a tremendous way in helping me heal myself and in turn help others learn how to help their own bodies heal.

We have twenty-four movable spinal segments in our spines called vertebra. Our skulls, which house the brain, the command center for our nervous systems, sits on top. Each set of two vertebra has a cartilage disc between them, which acts as a shock absorber and allows for spinal motion. Of course, then there is that triangular bone, called the sacrum, making up the center of our buttocks. Attached to either side of the sacrum are the two large, elephant-ear-shaped bones called ileums. This is where your leg bones attach, making up your hips. Your leg bones are connected to your hipbones. You remember Dad or Mom singing that to you years ago, right? At the very bottom of the spine, attached to the bottom end of your sacrum, are a string of several tiny bones called the coccyx.

The central nervous system travels along the spinal cord down a hole in the middle of the spinal column. This column is filled with liquid called cerebrospinal fluid, and it is housed in a glove-like sack. The spinal cord of the central nervous system breaks off into branches, which exit between each set of vertebrae. This is now called the peripheral nervous system, and it's on the periphery of the spinal column.

Amazingly enough, there are only thirty-one pairs of spinal nerves exiting the spinal column. These thirty-one nerves split and split again until all seventy-five trillion cells in the body have a nerve communicating back and forth with the brain – pretty crazy, right? I'm told that if you took everything away and left only the nerves, you'd still see the body standing there. What an amazing complex.

The reason I wanted to review the anatomy of the spine is so you can get an understanding of how many areas could be involved with your sciatic pain. This is the mechanical aspect, and anything here can contribute to the pain. You might consider what occurred when I fell out of the tree and crushed my bottom vertebra. Imagine stomping on a ham and cheese sandwich filled with lettuce and loaded with

mayonnaise; everything squishes together and gets distorted outward. Well, that is what happened to my spine. There are a lot of things affected here, and the compression to the nerves as they exited my lower back was causing a myriad of conditions. Not only did the part of the nerve that extends down my leg get affected, but so did the branch of that same nerve which controlled the function of my colon or large intestine. As a result of the disruption to this communication line between my brain and colon, all systems stopped. This is why Dr. York insisted I seek emergency medical help if that fateful adjustment had failed to work.

It's important to mention here that only 10 percent of your spinal nerve conveys pain. That means that 90 percent of the time the physiologic effects of spinal nerve disruption can go undiagnosed. As an example, if the segment of the nerve being disrupted is the track that goes to the colon, someone might suffer from IBS (Irritable Bowel Syndrome), colitis (inflammation of the colon), spastic colon, or who knows what while suffering no back pain.

Another branch of that same nerve track goes to the bladder. When there is disruption to this nerve, one might suffer from things like frequent bladder

infections or incontinence. The weakened immune response brought on by the decrease communication with the brain can allow opportunistic pathogens such as yeast (candida), bacteria, and others to take up residence in your body, causing all kinds of trouble. Of course, the typical handling for this is rounds of antibiotics and antifungals all of which destroy both the good and bad bacteria in not only the urinary track but also the whole body.

Let's not leave out the reproductive organs, which can be impacted, too. These same nerves are the major link between the brain and the sex organs. The penis, testis, and prostate for men and the ovaries, fallopian tubes, and vagina and all its parts for women.

There are many things that can go wrong with all these organs mentioned above, from dysmenorrhea (painful periods), to endometriosis (abnormal growth of the lining of the uterus), frequent bladder infections, colitis, irritable bowel syndrome, erectile dysfunction to incontinence. So often when patients come in for lower back pain and/or sciatica, I discover during the in-depth consultation that they are suffering from one or more of these disorders as well. The thing that is disappointing is that most of

the time, whoever was treating these patients prior to me, only treated the pain, and rarely asked about related organ dysfunction, nor explained the brain body connection. Instead, I find that the "specialist" put them on one or, often, a myriad of medications to hold down the symptoms. Dr. Jason Fung, nephrologist and bestselling author of *The Complete Guide to Fasting* and *The Obesity Code*, made this statement in an interview I did with him. He said, "If you could create a drug that wouldn't cure anyone but wouldn't kill them either, how long would they be on that drug?" Forever, seems to be the answer! Now multiply that by how many Americans take these types of meds. Wow, that's big business.

On April 20th 2015, AARP posted a statistic that the average forty-five-year-old takes four different prescription drugs every day. They revised the article December 6th 2017, stating, "Those aged 65 to 69 take an average of 15 prescriptions per year, while those from 80 to 84 take an average of 18, according to the American Association of Consultant Pharmacists.

"It gets worse. The AACP says that this practice – known as 'polypharmacy' – has a high price tag. The economic impact of medication-related problems

is estimated at $177.4 billion per year, rivaling that of Alzheimer's disease, cancer, diabetes and heart disease." These statistics speak for themselves, yet nothing is being done about it, except politicians arguing about how to get more and cheaper drugs into the hands of our citizens. Unbelievable!

Remember the basic tenet of chiropractic put forth by Dr. D.D. Palmer, is that "the power that made the body can heal the body." And in the words of the late great Dr. Reggie Gold, D.C., "The body needs no help, it just needs no interference."

Imagine how much healthier the citizens of our country would be if this was taught early on and practices of natural healing were a way of life? Now one thing about modern medicine is that it has advanced to an amazing degree and has saved an untold amount of lives, and thank God and modern science for that. We just need to stop the over-medication of our citizens. There is a better and healthier way.

Take both hands and hold them out in front of you like you are holding a basketball and rotate your hands in opposite directions. Imagine the five lower spinal bones or vertebrae, which make up the lumbar spine. These are attached to the sacrum, which

is attached to the coccyx. Now, you have the two elephant-ear-shaped bones attached to either side of the sacrum. These all have predicted motions given the movements of the body. Now, imagine an incredible complete matrix of pulleys, guide wires, temperature regulators, and governors, along with a lubricating system and communication system all regulated by a command center located far away up at the top of the spinal canal. When you twist the basketball one way or another, there are a lot of moving parts.

This concept of how the nerves exit the spine and control every single function of every cell and organ in the body is probably the single biggest misunderstanding people have regarding their bodies and how they operate and heal. How many times have I heard, "Why should I see a chiropractor? I'm not in pain!" Boy, this is such a huge misunderstanding forwarded by the drug pushers of the world that promote covering up all these symptoms with medications, but rarely, if ever, look up-stream for the actual cause of the problem.

After my fall out of that tree on Tightwad Hill, I developed asthma. Out of nowhere, I was suddenly afflicted with this very debilitating condition. It

wasn't until after a few adjustments with Dr. York that my asthma went away and never came back. When I mentioned this to Dr. York, he walked me to a spinal chart he had on the wall of his office and pointed to where the nerve in my upper back traveled to control my lungs. His thought was that when I landed in that seated position all those many years ago, the nerve in my upper back became somewhat entrapped as it exited the spine. Since I had so much pain from the lumbar injury, this secondary injury went relatively unnoticed.

So many times patients come in saying they were in a car accident ten plus years ago then start listing off all of their health conditions from migraines, numbness, chronic pains, or organ dysfunctions from A to Z. It is amazing how many times that just by looking at their x-rays, I can tell how old the injury is and even dictate some of their symptoms even before they express them to me.

Your nerves not only exit each set of vertebrae, but they also extend down through your sacrum and into and out of your coccyx bones. How many times have we fallen and landed on our butts, injuring these delicate bones and spinal nerves? Any injury that causes restriction to any aspect of this

mechanism can result in pressure on your nerves, contributing to sciatica and as mentioned above, any other body part or function associated with those nerves. By the way, you can have pressure on the spinal cord at any point in the spinal column, which can contribute to your lower back and sciatic pain. The nerve damage or miscommunication might even be in your neck or thoracic spine as in my case of asthma. There can be several mechanical malfunctions involved.

So, when a patient comes in and asks for a stretch or exercise to help their sciatic pain go away, it isn't that simple. Often times, the wrong thing to do is stretch; in fact, it can make things worse. Often, by the time people make their way into my office, they've already muddied the water pretty badly with all their potions, poisons, machines, and contraptions. Hopefully I get a chance to see them prior to things like surgery, nerve burning, or too many cortisone injections, but even then, there is a good chance they can still be helped. It takes a lot to understand the body's mechanics, as well as patience and years of experience to figure it out.

Many times, when I review the spinal x-rays with a patient and show an area of degenerative arthritis

to the patient, where the bones have slowly ground away the disc, making it look like a melted candle or worn out pencil eraser, the patient says, "I've never had an accident or injury." It's hard to imagine a forty, fifty, or sixty-year-old who never slipped or fell, who didn't play sports, and didn't have older siblings who used to love to use them as punching bags. Still, even sitting for a lifetime will wear out your spine.

At any rate, it is important to get a thorough spinal evaluation, including standing, full-spine x-rays, in order to determine which lifetime injuries, or even hereditary spinal defects, could be contributing to your condition. Not all chiropractors work off of x-rays, but I believe it's absolutely necessary, unless the doctor has x-ray vision or you are pregnant or have some other concern.

MRIs and CT scans are two types of imagery that can be helpful, especially if one suspects tumors, a fracture, infections, or bullets (of course, you cannot have an MRI if you have any metal in your body), but both of imagery these are taken lying down, which also distorts the findings. Bulging and herniated discs respond well to chiropractic with a skilled practitioner. I will speak about this more in a later chapter.

Chemical

The second side of the triangle is the chemical component, which is huge. This is where all the physiological operating systems come into play, but don't worry. I'll make it simple.

The definition of physiology is the branch of biology that deals with the normal functions or workings of living organisms and their parts. See, easy! So, what we are looking for here is anything that messes with the normal function of your body and its parts. There are a lot of contributing factors, and the three big ones are heavy metals, molds, and hidden infections.

There have been over 84,000 toxic chemicals dumped onto our planet since the early 1800s, and these toxins can cause a lot of problems, including inflaming the nerve and tissue surrounding the sciatic region of your body. These chemical poisons such as Glyphosate (or Roundup – we'll talk about this more later) and all the other herbicide and pesticide sprayed on the food we eat, the chemicals in products like Raid or your cosmetics, your soaps, cleaning detergent, and aluminum in your deodorant, let alone all the industrial chemical waste dumped into our air, earth and waterways can get

into your bodies and disrupt your hormone balance in the endocrine system. This can cause damage to the central and or peripheral nerves, or any of the organs and tissues of the body they get absorbed into. When the nervous system gets poisoned, even to a small degree, any condition and the symptoms associated with that condition could be amplified tremendously.

When looking for the cause of sciatic pain, or any bodily dysfunction, if one does not look for, and then eliminate or reduce, these damaging factors of toxicity, it is unlikely that true healing can occur. I will go into these issues further in a later chapter.

Mental

The last side of the pyramid is the mental or spiritual aspect. Most major medical textbooks state in their first few pages that psychosomatic causes exist to some degree in 95 percent of all disease, and this is huge. In a later chapter, we will delve into this in detail, but I want to make this clear, as I mentioned in Chapter 1, "If it's to be, it's up to me."

Fifteen years of drug addiction and having that druggie mindset (actually, barely having a mind at all at some points), taught me a lot about the mental

anguish, reasoning, and losses that come with the decision to either give up, stay sick, and/or, finally get well. I will dive into the mental gymnastics that stand in your way and what can be done about it in a future chapter, but for now, you can do it. I promise!

CHAPTER 4:

The Pinched Nerve, a Multifaceted Problem

Over the past thirty years, I've treated hundreds, if not thousands, of patients with sciatica or sciatic-type conditions. One thing that is common with almost all patients is that they believe that it just started two days prior or five years ago out of the blue. *I just woke up with it*, or *I've never had it before*, are pretty common thoughts. Sometimes, I hear people say, "It usually goes away in a few days, but this time it hasn't." This is usually followed by, "Can you give me a few stretches to do at home?" Oh, but only if it were that easy. Sometimes it is, but usually there are various complications, which have to be

taken into consideration if the patient truly wants to handle the situation permanently.

I remember a patient who came in about a year ago; he was a forklift driver and had been at it for about twenty years. Now, having been a forklift driver myself at one time, I understood the physical stresses put on his body. I know that more than half the time on a forklift you are turned backwards, making sure you don't run into anything. Right out of high school, I worked in a warehouse, which had smooth cement floors. Along with the bad lower back injury I suffered earlier in my life, I suffered from the constant twisting, not to mention the starting and stopping required while running the machine.

This guy worked for a local farmer and operated his forklift in a large storage barn with bumpy gravel. Perhaps you remember having your older brother or sister give you an "Indian rope burn," where they grabbed your forearm and twisted your skin with one hand in one direction, and the other hand in the other direction. The result is painful, but in the process, the twisting tightens up the skin, taking all the flexibility out of it. This is exactly what happens when a forklift driver turns his shoulder

backwards; he compresses the vertebra in his lower back, taking all of the shock-absorbing ability out of it. Now, as he drives backwards over that bumpy terrain, the shock absorbing disc pad goes under extreme pressure. This causes the disc to not only wear out quicker, kind of like a pencil eraser, but to also compress the spinal nerves.

On further questioning of his history, I discovered that he played Pop Warner football, then all the way through high school. His position was center, and he recalled several incidences where he'd had not only his bell rung but had also been knocked on his buttocks. He remembered being sore for a couple days, but that was it. As it was, he apparently had suffered many impacts at a young age to a point where his "green" bones had not had a chance to develop correctly. We call young bones "green," because at a young age they usually bend, rather than snap, under extreme physical impact.

"But it just started yesterday," people might say. However, what they don't understand is that yesterday's bumps were like the straws that broke the camel's back. I'm sure you have known somebody who developed a toothache "out of nowhere," but after a dentist examines their mouth and reviews

the x-rays, the dentist tells that person that they have a large cavity that has grown or expanded over time to the point where it finally hit the nerve. The dentist will tell this person that he thinks he can save the tooth by putting in a filling (hopefully, not mercury), a crown, or in worse cases a root canal or extraction.

Sometimes a patient might have an acute injury, a slip, or fall, or even a work or sporting accident. These can be easier to handle, but the danger is that the patient just wants to get out of pain, and once that happens, he forgets about the problem and goes back to his normal activities. If he is lucky, that will be the end of it.

An example of this type of injury can be understood by thinking about getting your finger slammed in a car door; we've probably all had that happen at one time in our lives. The result is a swollen, sore finger that throbs and is sore to the touch. This is exactly what happens in that acute injury. Given time, heat, ice, and some natural anti-inflammatories, you should feel better in a few days or weeks, but here is the danger if this happens too often – scar tissue forms, as with any injury. If the bones of the spine are not put through the proper motion as this

injury heals, the motion will be lost, and the process of "degeneration" begins.

So, now the patient goes about his business occasionally feeling stiff or even mild to moderate lower back and even leg pain. If he tries to ignore it, as most people do, he sets himself up for a potentially miserable future. Now, enter a series of "repetitive traumas" that could be as physical as sitting at a desk for eight to ten hours a day, working at a lumber yard, or in this patient's case, continuing to drive that forklift while twisted in an extreme posture. Eventually, he will end up in my office, and almost one for one, he will end up saying the six most common words I ever hear patients say when they finally come in, "I thought it would go away." If I had a nickel for every time I've heard those six words... but, actually, I am very happy that I did hear them, because I was able to help.

Degenerative Arthritis

This is a scary term and implies an old injury that didn't heal correctly and has now worn the disc so badly that even the bones or vertebra are starting to break apart. When this shows up on an x-ray, I know that this patient has had a history of back injuries,

small or large, and has handled the condition traditionally with painkillers. The worst thing that can happen is that the pain (symptoms) goes away, and they think they are healthy.

So often I hear these patients say, "Well, I used to have back pain, but that was twenty years ago," or, "Aww, it just comes and goes. My doctor prescribed ibuprofen for the symptoms." When I ask how often they take painkillers, they often say, "Oh, usually I only need two a day, sometimes four." I ask them if they ever read the back of the bottle, where it says, "Only take for fifteen days, then consult a physician." They shrug their shoulders and say, "He didn't really recommend anything else."

I have one patient, named Dean, who is in his late fifties. I met him in a business group I am a part of, and I'd known him for about six months when he finally made his way into my office. The thing was, Dean wasn't there for pain, but his wife had enrolled him in a nutritional workshop I conducted that was designed to reduce inflammation and increase energy (more on this later).

Well, after only three weeks on the program, I asked how everyone was doing. Dean raised his hand and said, "I'm off all the ibuprofen I've been

taking." The rest of the class applauded with their support. When I asked Dean how many he was taking and for how long, he said that he had been taking up to forty 800 mg ibuprofen a week, and that he had been doing that for years. The body's major organs that can be affected by ibuprofen are the liver and kidneys, and this can raise blood pressure as well. However, it is the slow, steady destruction that usually takes its toll, with chronic inflammation and degeneration of the blood vessels, brain, liver, kidneys, etc.

I'm sorry to tell you that this is more common than one might think. We live in a "supersize" world, and most of us operate on, "If two is good, four must be better." Further, most of us never think that we will be the ones to develop such problems – until we do. As an example, think about how many times you've slowly inched your way up to, and past, a car accident. Everyone looks on with a blank stare and maybe makes a comment under their breath or says a little prayer for the victims usually not ever putting themselves in victim's position.

When I heard what Dean said, my jaw dropped. It was amazing that he was still alive. The maximum recommended dose of ibuprofen for adults

is 1,200 mg, and Dean was regularly taking 4,570 mg, almost four times the safe dosage. Dean changed his diet, lost thirty-five pounds, lost the inflamed look in his face and body, and looked at least twenty years younger. What is even more amazing is seeing examples like this happen again and again as people work their way through the processes and tools in this book.

Let's revisit the comment, "The pain used to bother me, but not anymore." Too often when I look at weight-bearing x-rays, meaning they are taken when a patient stands so that gravity is in play, I see thin lower back discs and bones covered with spurs. Spurs are like callouses on your hands from working with a hammer or garden tool too long. However, the difference is that these callouses on the vertebra are made of bone and they don't go away like those on your hands. This tells me that this condition started anywhere from five to ten, or even thirty years ago. Sometimes, I can see that it is even a genetic defect that started in utero. You can make a pretty good educated guess of when the accident or injury occurred when you've looked at as many x-rays as I have. In the thirty-plus years I've been in practice, I've reviewed over 30,000 sets of x-rays, all

including those of the lumbar spine. In fact, one day I added it up just for fun, since I typically take seven different views of each patient, and the count was about 200,000 individual x-rays. That is a lot of film.

No offense to your family medical doctor, but when you go in to see him for any spinal issues or neurological problems, ask him how many sets of x-rays he's reviewed. The answer will most likely be "very few" because a non-treating radiologist usually reads all the x-rays and then sends a report to the family doctor. The point here is that your family doctor specializes in infections, cuts, viruses, and medications. Someone needs to be that guy and thank God for them! However, you should understand that the typical medical doctor gets less than 115 hours of x-ray training in school, whereas chiropractors get about 360 hours of the same training. Still, it is not about the training in school; it's about practical experience in the field.

Beyond the practical experience of reading thousands of x-rays in a clinical setting, a family doctor's typical solution for sciatica is drugs and physical therapy. Sometimes this works, but most often I hear, "They just gave me exercises." This is a big problem for several reasons. For one, if there is an

underlying injury, and there usually is, then once the "symptoms" go away, the patient is released without any evaluation of the normal function of the spinal segments. This is a big oversight and is what typically drives patients into my office. Just like a tiny cavity can turn into a root canal, a minor "sprain strain" can turn into a degenerative, or, if not caught in time, a fused disc. Hopefully, we catch it before it fuses, but even if it has, remember there are another twenty-three vertebra to protect from premature destruction from improper motion and altered nerve function.

People may not be aware of a chiropractor's education in comparison to that of a medical doctor, so I included this chart from Cleveland College of Chiropractic (which can be accessed at https://biology.uni.edu/sites/default/files/chiropractic_education_vs_medical_education.pdf) to show where a chiropractor's training is concentrated.

Comparison of Overall Curriculum Structure

Characteristics	Chiropractic Schools		Medical Schools	
	Average	Percentage	Average	Percentage
Total Contact Hours	4826	100	4667	100
Basic Sciences Hours	1420	29	1200	26
Clinical Sciences Hours	3406	71	3467	76
Chiropractic Sciences Hours	1975	41	N/A	N/A
Clerkship	1405	29	3467	76

Chiropractic vs. Medical

Chiropractic	Subject	Medical
540	Anatomy-Physiology	508
240	Physiology	326
360	Pathology-Geriatrics-Pediatrics	401
165	Chemistry	325
120	Microbiology	114
630	Diagnosis, Dermatology, Ears, Eyes, Nose, Throat	324
320	Neurology	112
360	Radiology	148
60	Psychology-Psychiatry	144
60	Obstetrics-Gynecology	148
310	Orthopedics	156
3065	**Total**	**2706**

People often say, "Oh, my doctor said it is normal wear and tear; it's just old age." That couldn't be further from the truth, I say.

If you bought a set of brand-new Michelin tires (which I also used to sell for nine years), and then after the 20,000-mile mark, the right front tire was worn out on the outside only, would that be "normal" wear and tear? I think not. And don't blame your spouse for hitting the curb while parking, you know it was you! Anyway, if you went back to the tire salesman for a warranty, he'd just laugh. This is the same as your spine. When you have one or two pair of spinal vertebra that have worn out faster than the rest of your spine, it is not normal wear and tear; it is advancing degenerative arthritis caused by misaligned vertebra or subluxations, from anything like an old sports injury, childhood slip and fall, or even a work-related condition brought on from sitting on your fanny for eight hours a day, and oh yeah, don't forget about the time you sit commuting to work an hour each way.

Sitting is probably the biggest hidden contributor to lower back pain and sciatica. Why? This is because when you sit all day, every day, the discs between your vertebra usually get their nutrition

through a process called imbibing or drinking. This occurs with motion, which kind of massages the cartilaginous discs, keeping them thick and healthy. The cartilage cells are called chondrocytes and newer research has proven that these chondrocytes can continue to produce and divide. This only happens under healthy circumstances, such as proper joint function, lack of cellular or global inflammation, and proper nutrition, and as people rarely live under perfect health conditions, sciatica develops.

Is Surgery My Only Option?

About a year ago, a couple long-time patients of mine asked if I thought I could help their co-worker. When I asked about her situation, they told me she was lifting something and had severe low back pain. They said she had been on her back for several days and that they wanted to get her in. I asked them to send her in, so that I would do a complimentary consultation with her (which is my usual practice). When Carol came into the office, she looked miserable. She was using a walker and could barely move. She was an attractive woman in her fifties, and about thirty pounds overweight.

She told me that she had just left the emergency room at the local hospital where they had done an MRI. She was told that she had a severely herniated disc and needed immediate surgery. Luckily for her, the surgeon would not be in until the following Monday. It was a Wednesday, so I had some work to do. After a thorough consultation, I discovered that she had grown up on a farm in the Midwest. She had been active as a kid and was somewhat of a tomboy. She remembered many injuries as a kid and was even told that she had broken her tailbone when she fell off a horse. For the past twenty years, Carol had a desk job and had lost her athletic body.

The examination revealed severe inflammation at the lower lumbar level. I told her I needed a set of standing spinal x-rays, and when she asked if the MRI was good enough, I explained that MRIs are taken lying down and often distort things. She said she understood and was agreeable. The full spine x-ray showed that she was leaning far over to the left side, putting much more weight on the left side of her body.

"But my sciatica is on my left side, that doesn't make sense," Carol said.

"Right," I agreed. If I had a nail in my left shoe, I would typically lean away from the nail, not put more weight on that foot. I could see her questioning, and then understanding, as I began to explain what was happening to her.

I explained that the nervous system was so confused because of the extreme inflammation around the nerve, the herniated disc, and with the effects of the Demerol shot they gave her in her butt that her body didn't know what to do. I could see a glimmer of hope develop in her eyes and a softness embrace her cheeks. I remember her grasping my hand trembling, "Can you help me, Doctor? I'm afraid of surgery, but they told me I needed it." Carol had never been to a chiropractor before and, as a rule, didn't like doctors.

I continued to explain her x-ray's findings and then told her that there was a good chance I could help her, but it would be important that she do everything I asked of her.

She sat for a minute and then said, "I trust you, Doctor; please, what do I need to do?" Now, it is quite something to have someone in so much pain and so desperate to grant you their trust. This is an amazing privilege and one of the things I cherish.

I explained what I was going to do. Now, a lot of chiropractors I know would not attempt what I did, but I knew that if I could get some pressure off her lumbar nerve, I had a chance of relieving her sciatica to some degree. After all, this is what Dr. York did for me some forty-five years ago. I also told her what Dr. York told me, and Carol told me that she had been constipated and was having trouble holding her urine, so I knew there was a tremendous amount of pressure, not only on the sciatic nerve, which went down her leg, but also pressure affecting the organ function.

This was a serious condition, so I told her, "I am going to try to move the bone off of your nerve. It may hurt a bit (that is not always the case, it just usually gives relief), kind of like taking glass out of your finger, but if I can get it to move, you should feel some relief soon. However, if I can't get it to move, I'm going to ask that you go back to the emergency room and let them know about your bowel and bladder condition." Carol agreed, so I began the procedure.

Again, this is something I do because of my years of experience. I can't even tell you how many chiropractic interns have come to work for me over

the years and look on in horror as I do what I was about to do. I don't understand their shock, as chiropractic, which was discovered in 1895, was established on the principle that the body has the ability to heal itself and that if you can free up the nerve and re-establish correct communication, it can do just that. This concept goes all the way back to Hippocrates, yet these poor students come out of chiropractic school afraid to adjust, but I will talk more on that later.

Once I got Carol's agreement, I helped her onto her side with her left side up. She was clearly in severe pain, no matter what position she was in. First, I did a seldom-used technique and released the meningeal sheath, a glove-like sheath that houses the spinal cord and stops the spinal fluid from leaking out. Imagine holding a sheet of cellophane, stretching it between your two hands. Now, twist it one way or the other, and you will find that there are stressors along the cellophane, some tighter than others. Almost every time there is a spinal injury, including disc injuries; this type of stress is put on the spine. After about five minutes of this technique, I could feel Carol begin to relax and it felt like the time was right to move the bone.

I got Carol in the correct position so that there would be little resistance to the chiropractic adjustment. Having a thorough understanding of what is called the biodynamics of the spine, or the proper motions of the spine (how the body's joints are supposed to move), is something only a skilled chiropractor will be able to do to make a correction with certainty.

So, I positioned Carol correctly on the adjusting table, asked her to take a breath in, let it out, and relax her upper shoulder backwards. Then, I produced an exactly calculated motion on a specific part of the fifth or bottom vertebra. There was a loud pop and Carol exclaimed. I could feel the heat rush to her skin as the sympathetic surge of adrenaline flowed through her body.

I remember her just lying there, sideways on the table, as she burst into tears. Carol started sobbing, and it was hard for me to refrain from crying as well; even now, recalling the moment fills my eyes with tears. I had been at this long enough to feel the relief in her body and to sense the muscle start to relax; the adjustment was a success. I took a moment to thank God, and then thought about

how Dr. Anthony York had performed almost the exact procedure on me all those many years ago.

Once Carol was ready, I helped her to her feet. I'll never forget the look on her face when she realized that she could put weight on her legs without the support of the walker. I instructed her to take it easy, recommended that she consider not taking painkillers so that her body could sense what was happening, and to go home and come back the next day. As Carol made her way up the aisle to the front desk, she continued to cry and say, "thank you," over and over again. I know that her body would do the healing; I had just helped remove the interference. How many patients don't get this chance? How many people end up in surgery or addicted to deadly drugs like the opioids that plague our country?

Carol went on to do my recommendations. I taught her how to handle the chronic inflammation in her body through dietary changes and cellular detoxification. Carol lost thirty pounds and even surprised us one day when she walked into the office excited, telling us that she'd been asked out on a date. Again, I'm getting filled with goosebumps as I relate this. Carol was an attractive woman when I first met her, but after cleaning up her diet, losing

thirty pounds, and getting a healthy glow about her, she not only looked twenty years younger, but was also stunning.

Subluxation: The Bigger Picture

The main thing to understand here is that the lack of symptoms does not mean you are healthy. Think about the everyday "Joe," seemingly perfectly healthy, who dies suddenly of a heart attack, or "Sally," who just comes down with cancer. No, these issues have been brewing for a long time. Remember, pain is there to let you know that something is wrong. Unfortunately, sometimes the pain nerve just goes numb after a while, and you forget about or ignore the problem. My concern here is often times the symptoms may not present as pain but rather as other conditions related to organs or system dysfunction. These "dis-eases" may be treated medically with drugs to mask the symptoms, thus leaving an underlying condition to develop. It is important to remember the three aspects of health here: physical, chemical and emotional. All of these can have ill effects on the body, resulting in the development of chronic disease. However, I should point out, all three aspects can

have amazingly healthful effects as well; we just need to learn to use and nurture them.

As an example, our bodies are an adaptive organism. We don't feel the clothes we wear after a while or the rings on our fingers. In the same way, your body will eventually shut off pains, minor or major, so you can get on with the business of living. However, the problem is that when left unhandled, these issues come back with a vengeance and disrupt, and sometimes even consume, your life. Don't let that happen to you or someone you love – find help.

Rest assured that your ability to assume a causative viewpoint regarding your health and well-being has everything to do with you understanding a bit more about how the body has the ability to heal itself. Your body's health is greatly influenced by how toxins tear down the foundation of your immune system and its ability to handle the plethora of toxins it is exposed to from the environment. The next chapter will help you understand what role toxins play in your health and give you solutions to help reduce their effect.

CHAPTER 5:

Toxic Inflammation

It seems that almost any magazine you pick up lately has the words "chronic inflammation" on the cover and addresses its role in chronic disease. This is an important topic for us to understand as we look to eliminate the various factors involved with sciatica.

With that being said, so began the war on inflammation. Heart disease, arthritis, colitis, gastritis, dementia, diabetes, and even hormone imbalances are being linked to chronic inflammation. In fact, age-related disease is the biggie when talking about chronic inflammation; it can all be linked to chronic inflammation. A recent study from the University of Michigan stated that over eighty-one million Americans suffer from multiple chronic diseases,

meaning three or more. A chronic disease is defined as a condition, which lasts more than three months. Eighty-one million Americans makes up about one quarter of our population, but where is this inflammation located, what is causing it, and can it be reversed?

This is a great question, and I'm glad you asked! It's about time somebody did. Here is what I mean. Western medicine is fantastic for emergency medicine, and if I break a bone or cut myself to the point where I can't glue it together with superglue, I'm the first person to seek out the great medical system we have. However, when it comes to getting my body healthy and keeping it healthy, I found after years of suffering with severe and sometimes debilitating pain, that, "if it's to be, it's up to me."

So, here is my point. If chronic disease is created by chronic inflammation, do we keep chasing chronic inflammation around and around the mulberry bush until our bodies give out, or might we step back for a minute and try to figure out what causes chronic inflammation?

Well, that has been done, and to our surprise, the answer was right in front of us for years: chronic inflammation is caused by toxins. Toxins take many

forms; they can come from the foods we eat, the air we breathe, the water we drink, the clothes we wear, or the products we put on our body, and now we found out they can be and are passed down through our dear mom's umbilical blood. Gee, thanks mom! As you will remember, toxins make up the chemical portion of the health triangle. In the next section I will discuss how specifically these toxins interact with us in our daily lives.

Glyphosate, the Widow Maker

One of the biggest safety issues for Americans regarding foods is Monsanto's glyphosate. I imagine you've heard of Monsanto by now, but if not, glyphosate or Roundup is sprayed directly on the grain crops of America's farms as well as some other countries around the world. The company has actually created a gene that is glyphosate resistant and inserted it in the DNA sequence of plants. This way they can spray the crops liberally just prior to harvest. This allows the green foliage to dry up but doesn't kill the plant. They yield a bigger harvest by doing this. Also, the other non-modified plants that may grow in the fields are killed while the glyphosate resistant crop plants remain stable. There is

no nutritional value in the use of Roundup aka glyphosate. It just makes Monsanto more money at the expense of our health. Thank God some companies such as Costco are refusing to carry the planet-killing product anymore.

The article "Almost all Americans Are Contaminated with Glyphosate Herbicide" published by *Health Impact News* estimates the global usage of glyphosate. It states, "18.9 billion pounds have been used globally since its introduction in 1974, making it the most widely and heavily applied weed-killer in the history of chemical agriculture." It is very sad knowing the horrific damage glyphosate has caused, not only to us humans but to the earth's microbiome, the microbes which even help the plant's absorb nutrients.

This product has not only been linked to several kinds of cancer, but it is also a huge contributor to a multitude of health conditions. Primarily, it virtually destroys the gut membrane separating the contents of the intestinal track from the blood stream. It opens up the "tight junctions," allowing larger undigested food particles as well as opportunistic pathogens to enter the body. This and the myriad of hormones like estrogens and growth hormones

injected into our feed animals, along with the other pesticides, herbicides, fungicides, additives, and fillers allowed by the Food and Drug Administration (13,000 of them) are slowly destroying our immune systems and all other systems in our bodies. These same toxins also break down something called the BBB or Blood Brain Barrier, allowing heavy metals like mercury and lead as well as all these other toxic chemicals to enter the brain, causing damage that manifests as things like dementia, Alzheimer's, Parkinson's and even brain cancer.

Let's look at the bigger picture, though. If glyphosate can cause cancer, what about those of us who don't contract cancer (which I will discuss later), but develop all kinds of different, chronic conditions? What is it that glyphosate is doing anyway? That is another good question. According to Dr. Stephanie Seneff, a senior research scientist at MIT, the abrupt rise in almost all chronic disease is in direct ratio to the rise in usage of glyphosate. When she presented this to a senate subcommittee a few years ago, there was little interest. She states in her paper dated December 2013 titled "Glyphosate – Pathways to Modern Disease" that many conditions have increased in direct ratio to the usage of glyphosate

on our crops. Besides the aforementioned damage to the gut, she suggests that diseases such as Alzheimer's, Parkinson's, infertility, kidney, and liver disease and even death can be the result of glyphosate exposure. Seneff asked the question, how many people would suffer before this product and others like it are abolished? Suffice it to say, the non-organic grains grown in this country should be avoided altogether; they are toxic. As of this writing, Monsanto has been busted and both it and its parent company Bayer have been sued for hundreds of millions of dollars.

But hold on, don't close the book here. Since the publication of Seneff's article, the jury is out, and the verdict is in. Monsanto was found guilty of lying and withholding evidence during their trial, which proved they knew that glyphosate is a carcinogenic substance that they poured gallons by the billions of into the environment.

Is the FDA Food and Drug Administration Guilty of Treason?

How many other chemicals end up getting into our bodies that shouldn't? Wow, this is a great question I don't have an answer to, but I'm sure it's a huge

number. The intestinal wall is designed to allow only certain nutrients such as vitamins, nutrients, fatty acids, and amino acids into the blood stream so that we can feed our cells the nutrients necessary to sustain life. Remember, inflammation of the intestines, such as colitis, Crohn's disease, diverticulitis, or even gastritis, allow many opportunistic pathogens to enter into the body and take up a stronghold so they can wreak havoc on our bodies. This can manifest as chronic infection, inflammation, and even organ failure. Today colorectal cancer is the third most common diagnosis in the US.

Those of us who've lived for a while remember the 1960s and 70s and the beginning of the organic food generation. Well, since then, the reasons to move towards the organic way of life is one-hundred-fold. We now live in the most toxic time in human history; man has made over 84,000 chemicals that have been released onto the planet. In fact, most of these chemicals have not been tested for their safety or for their short- or long-term effects on the environment.

Looking at the food we eat, I think my sister, Sudi, said it best. Years ago, she made a statement that stuck with me. She stated that the Food and Drug

Administration (FDA) is treasonous when it comes to protecting the citizens of the United States from the harmful effects of food toxicity. The definition she used for treason was "betrayal after trust." We've put our trust in the FDA's ability to keep our food safe, yet they have allowed billions of pounds of these toxins be released into the atmosphere and into the food we eat.

Our cell membrane is the source of our innate intelligence. Dr. Bruce Lipton, stem cell biologist and bestselling author of *The Biology of Belief*, states in his famous video "Our Cell Membrane Can Change Our DNA" (you can watch the video here: https://www.youtube.com/watch?v=5e8vB7AdcWI) that if you take a healthy cell and put it in an adverse environment, the cell will immediately start to die. If you take the same cell and move it to a healthy environment, it will start to flourish. In other words, this tells us that if we want to live long and prosper, we better start cleaning up our environment – both internal and external.

Black Sabbath and Other Heavy Metals

Other factors which work in concert with glyphosate and other toxins are something known as heavy

metals, and I ain't talking about Black Sabbath. Heavy metals are abundant in our current environment, and we are exposed to many of them each day in staggering doses. If that isn't bad enough, Dr. Michael Skinner, an epidemiologist, says the lion's share (over four generations worth) of heavy metals are actually passed down to us through our mothers' umbilical blood. In fact, the number one source of lead is Mom – thanks, Mom. Lead is attracted to, and stored in, our bones.

Lead actually competes with calcium and has a stronger binding capacity than calcium, so it often displaces calcium in the body. Lead accumulates in your body where calcium is usually stored, such as your bones. Lead has deleterious effects on the brain and nervous system. It also affects the heart and blood vessels adversely. The kidneys, the digestive and reproductive systems are also damaged by lead. A list of symptoms such as depression, anxiety, as well as certain organ failure can all be linked to the accumulation of lead in your system.

The point here is that when Mom incubates her baby, all of the best parts of her are sacrificed for the development of the fetus. Since lead is stored in Mom's bones, as calcium is being called up for

transfer, so is lead. The most obvious mental symptoms of lead poisoning are depression and anxiety. Not only do we get this lead dosage from Mom, but we are also bombarded with it in today's toxic world.

The second most abundant toxic metal, and in fact, probably the most toxic of all, is mercury. We get this from so many sources, and for years, our exposure to this extremely toxic substance went unchecked. Silver fillings are 50 percent mercury, and for a long time, the dental industry stuck this within inches of our brains. We were told, and still are, that it is safe, but I recommend you start looking at the real facts. Mercury has been used for 150 years in dental fillings, so what this means is that the majority of our mercury is because of good old Mom. Again, thanks, Mom!

The controversy goes on and on, but I'll tell you this, if you look up the top symptoms of mercury toxicity, you'll find symptoms such as anxiety, nervousness, irritability or mood swings, memory problems, depression, numbness and even physical tremors. I think it is terrible that a majority of our children are receiving mind altering medications for things like depression or anxiety without even giving consideration to or investigating their heavy

metal toxic load. I believe this oversight smacks of negligence.

Okay, back to sciatica. The deal with heavy metals in your body is that they love to accumulate in the worst of all places; heavy metals love the brain and especially the endocrine system, or specifically the hypothalamus and pituitary glands. These heavy metals also hang out in major organs, such as the liver and kidneys. Even worse is that they cross through the cell wall and enter into the cell body and even the mitochondria.

If we were only worried about the heavy metals, it would be one thing, but it's not. Heavy metals make the bed for other dangerous neuropathologic opportunists, changing the pH of our tissue and making a more welcoming environment for pathogens, such as molds, viruses, bacteria, and even parasites to nest and multiply.

So, what does this have to do with my sciatica, you ask? Well, remember that favorite villain, chronic inflammation? Well, that is the result of these unwelcome guests in our bodies' tissue. Now, a lot of us no longer possess a strong immune system, but even if we did, these bad guys are hard at work to create that dreaded phrase, "age-related disease."

However, to the sciatic sufferer, this dictates localized inflammation over and around an already inflamed area. The more inflamed our body is, the worse any problem will manifest – especially sciatic problems.

Before writing this, I was talking to my best friend, Bill, you remember, the same guy who was with me when I fell out of the tree. We've been best friends ever since he and his twin brother Andy crashed my fifth birthday party many, many years ago. Bill became a medical doctor and while in the military was deployed as a military doctor over seventeen times. He has seen his fair share of sciatica and related what you already know. When sciatica is bad, it's so debilitating and painful that even morphine barely touches it. As an emergency doctor, Bill's main goal is to relieve his patients' pain. I understand that pain and I want to help you get your pain handled as soon as possible; however, my goal is to also ensure that you are equipped with the know-how to make sure your sciatica doesn't come back!

There's Mold in Them-Thar-Hills

Molds and hidden infections are two more issues that go overlooked, and if not searched for and

handled, could leave you suffering needlessly into the future. It is everywhere, and when someone is exposed to it, he or she can have a boatload of trouble getting rid of it because when mold takes a hold, it won't let go.

Mold even has its own passage in the Bible. In Leviticus 14, God told Moses to inspect the house for mildew. If he found it, he was to get a priest to come and inspect it. If the priest suspected bad mold, he would have Moses get it removed and disposed. God was very clear that after seven days the priest was to reinspect for mildew. If he found the mildew again, the house was to be torn down, the timbers and any furniture or clothing in the house was to be burned, and any stones buried deep and away from town.

Mold is tenacious and takes a strong hold in and on the body. It persists, but do not despair. I can help. A little later, I'll talk more about how to handle mold.

There is an amazing test available today from Vibrant America. It is the only lab test that looks for thirty-one different molds. When it's time to dig into the causes of your condition this may be an appropriate tool. There is a neurotoxic questionnaire that you can find at www.mccollumwellness.com. By filling this out and sending it to my office,

I can help you determine if some part of your condition is mold related. If so, I can help guide you through the most current techniques in handling mold in your body. And by the way, because of new research continually emerging, mold protocols are updated regularly to be the most effective.

Hidden Infections: Underlying Cause to Many Health Conditions?

Hidden infections are an amazingly overlooked condition across the board when one suffers from a chronic disease, whether sciatica or some other condition. The source of these hidden infections could fool you. I'd been working with a young lady for about six months, trying to help her with some chronic conditions; she was not in good shape. We worked on everything from diet, to heavy metal detoxification, to intermittent fasting, and the ketogenic diet. She even had a kidney infection that would not respond to nutrition or antibiotics, so she had to have surgical intervention. Finally, I introduced her to a biological dentist in town, recommending she get what is called a cone-beam or three-dimensional x-ray of her mouth, which is essentially a CAT scan of her jaw. As I suspected, she

had a terrible hidden infection deep in her jawbone at the spot of extraction of one of her wisdom teeth, which was pulled many years earlier. These "cavitations" are more common than one might think and can develop in root canals or even as in her case at the sight of old tooth extractions.

There is a ligament that holds the tooth in its socket called the periodontal ligament. Often times, when there is an extraction, this ligament is neglected. As the gum heals over, this ligament dies in the wound and then basically rots or necroses buried deep in the jawbone. This creates an unhealthy environment perfect for those opportunistic pathogens to make their beds, and they do. Recently, I saw the pathology reports of two patients; one was the woman I was just speaking of and the other was of a colleague who was having health issues. Both of them had at least eight highly dangerous bacteria well above the "safe" level that had taken up residence in these lesions.

These cavitations and their occupants start to create a manufacturing plant of "mycotoxins," which are basically the excretions or byproducts (poop) of these bacterial, mold, and viral beasts, which are slowly and clandestinely excreted into

your body's lymph system. These toxins amplify any condition you have and even work to alter the genes in your cells turning on bad things such as cancers, Alzheimer's disease, and Parkinson's disease to name a few. When our genes get altered, a myriad of "age-related diseases" can develop. To the point of this subject of sciatica, any of these inflammatory situations will increase the symptoms of pain due to the irritability of the toxin on the body's tissue.

If you suspect you might have cavitations, have patience. The worst thing you could do is try to correct them without first dumping a huge amount of the toxins out of your bucket first. It is imperative that you detox correctly and thoroughly before adding more toxins into your circulatory system. Because of the viruses, bacteria, molds, Lyme, and other pests that reside in your mouth the cavitations can be very virulent, you must take precautions. Imagine finding a mouse nest in your garage. If you disturb it, the mice scurry away to the next best hiding place until they feel safe enough to emerge. This is exactly what these pathogens do once evicted from their comfortable home. And believe me, these things can make you very sick.

And if you are already in a bad way, this could push you over the edge. Please contact me if you feel like you need help with this.

Sciatica and Our Toxic World

If you desire to truly get rid of your sciatic condition, it is essential that you explore the world of toxicity as it relates to you, your sciatica, and the future of your well-being. There are several tests and studies you can seek out in order to discover your toxic load and even the possible existence of hidden infections in your body. I list these a little further on, but I caution you to understand that there is an exact sequence in which these should be addressed so as not to create even more problems by unnecessarily unleashing and spreading these toxins throughout your already compromised body.

We can assume that you are toxic, we all are, it's just a matter of how full is your cup? I will offer many suggestions on how to go about fixing all this in a later chapter, but suffice it to say, start by eliminating all foods that are not organic, including meats, all GMOs and any foods that didn't come from the dirt. What I mean by this is any processed foods are not real foods and remember that the FDA has

allowed over 13,000 additive and fillers be added to these processed foods. Yuck!

So if you pick up a box, package, or can of any foodstuff that has words on it you can't pronounce or define, put it down and *run for your life*. Because it depends on it.

Stay away from all sugars, white flours, American grown grains of any kind, breads, sodas, fruit juices, and cereals. Sorry but these are loaded with sugar, and if you value your health, you will have to move in this direction. In one of the classes I will introduce in a bit, you will learn an easy, step-by-step procedure, which will actually make this doable and relatively easy to accomplish.

I'm hoping you are starting to see that it's not just about relieving the pain – pain relief is just the beginning. Health and well-being are so much more about being excited about living. Your future is bright, and I only hope I can help you on your journey!

CHAPTER 6:

Firing Your Boss and Other Troublemakers

Sometimes our best friends are our worst enemies. I'm sure you've heard the American-English idiom: "Can't see your nose in front of your face." The meaning here is being oblivious to something obvious and in clear view. Have you ever noticed your friends or family members being a victim of this phrase? Perhaps you've noticed that this has affected you as well; I certainly have. In fact, there is no doubt that I am missing some obvious circumstances as I write this book. In this chapter, I will outline the not-so-obvious troublemakers in your life that may be impacting your life.

Psychosomatic Illness, How Your Mind Can Affect Your Health

Looking back at the all too well known, but not so understood, health pyramid, we find that its sides consist of physical, chemical, and emotional/spiritual elements. Any medical textbook you pick up undoubtedly has a statement in the beginning commenting on the fact that nearly 95 percent of all disease and malaise in our modern world has some kind of stressor at its source. It will go on to state that this same 95 percent can be caused by mental stress. This has been understood since the dawn of modern thinking. A good example of this is when a person develops a bleeding ulcer from worry. Stomach acids can be so strong that if there is nothing in the stomach to digest, it digests the walls of your stomach; this is crazy but true. The pH, or acid level, of the gastric acid or hydrochloric acid produced by the parietal cells or epithelial cells in your stomach is a pH of two, which can eat a hole in your wooden countertop.

When your body is under the effect of mental stressors, your health is affected. I'm sure you've heard of the hormone cortisol – the stress hormone. This hormone is useful in many ways for our bodies.

Because most bodily cells have cortisol receptors, this hormone affects many different functions in the body. Cortisol can help control blood sugar levels, regulate metabolism, reduce inflammation, and assist with memory formulation. It also has a controlling effect on salt and water balance and helps control blood pressure. Cortisol is often called the body's built-in alarm system. It is excreted into the blood stream from the outer layer, or cortex, of our adrenal glands, (adrenal glands are small almond sized glands that sit on top of our kidneys) in response to a perceived danger. It is this hormone that gives Mom the superpower to pick up a car to pull her baby out from underneath after an accident, and it is also excreted in times of injury or danger to help you run for your life. In the animal kingdom, this hormone has served in survival, allowing prey to flee predators and lambs to escape lions.

When it comes to sentient beings, we run into a problem. Since we have the ability to reason, which is a trait one could argue that lower animals may not have, we tend to overthink things, either consciously or unconsciously. It is not my purpose to solve the problems of the mind here, but rather to point out how perceived stress is a potential and

real threat to our health and well-being. This mental stress can manifest in many ways:

The Stress from School Days

The hierarchy in school is a good example of this. Have you ever looked at the social mechanics of our children and what they go through in school? Our children are exposed to so much mental stress, either by their peers or the struggling learning system they confront. The number of children put on mind-altering drugs is astounding. Anxiety and depression are at epidemic levels, yet rather than looking for up-stream causes, like the heavy metals such as lead and mercury or looking at the state of the child's digestive system (90 percent of our serotonin receptors exist in our digestive tracts), children are just prescribed chemical handcuffs. Any attempts at truly looking up-stream, to chemical and even physical stressors, such as pressure on the brain stem, are only rarely considered.

In addition, often times, the friends we hang out with are condescending, either overtly, or even worse, covertly. So many great artists were taken down by their well-meaning friends – look at Michael Jackson, Billy Holiday, Whitney Huston,

Otis Redding, and more. However, when these bullies don't literally take our lives, they work to demean us and discourage our ability to reach for the stars.

Constant Negative News

Finally, the news media and the sensationalists love to report that the sky is falling. It has too many people living in a perceived dangerous environment.

In recent history some countries or regimes have artificially set up crises, to keep their population enslaved and in fear. How many times in the history of the human race has some dictator, or other faction, suppressed a populous into slavery of the mind or body? Suppressive regime's like Hitler's Germany, China's Mao Zedong, have made the citizens of earth fearful for their lives. This kind of fear, often sensationalized by the media, can have a huge effect on our health.

The best and easiest example I can think of for being mentally enslaved is the phrase "he was drowning on dry land," or, "she was drowning in shallow water, when all she had to do was stand up." It's a lot like the question "Is your cup half-empty or half-full?" I believe we can actually train ourselves

to perceive the half-full concept. I heard a phrase many years ago which stuck with me. It took years for me to manifest this concept, but it has finally sunk in. That phrase is, "You will be the same person in five years as you are today except for the people you meet and the books you read." The first thing that must happen is for the individual to decide. Sometimes this comes from disaster, severe injury or loss. Once the decision is made, it is important to find the tools that most resonate with you to move forward.

Anguish for Those You Love

The mental handicap of being mentally enslaved can be worse than any virus ever known or any dictator who ever walked this earth. The question is – how do we get our loved ones out of this trap? I've seen so many moms and dads devastated as their sons and daughters fall victim to the drug epidemic that has stolen so many lives. Having somehow pulled myself out of this terrible addictive lifestyle, I look on with anguish as parents sacrifice all that they have to save their children.

Here is a true-life example I have lived through regarding the devastating effects of mental stress

on a person's health. When I was ten years old, my sixteen-year-old older brother, decided "the world is just not ready for me" and took his own life. My parents, who never got along at all anyway, berated him for his inability to study, who he hung out with, and who knows what else. Finally, because of several factors we'll never know, my brother, AJ, gave up.

My mother was devastated, as were we all. Outwardly, she blamed my dad – privately and publicly. However, in reality, she never forgave herself. She was an amazing artist and taught classes to the doctors at the local hospital in the ballroom of our Berkeley home. As a kid, I watched her paint and observed how the beautiful Monet-type landscapes slowly evolved into troubled abstract expressions of her eternal pain.

One evening many years after the fact, I lined up twenty plus years of her work in my living room and played Maurice Ravels' brilliant rendition of composer Modest Mussorgsky's masterpiece, *Pictures at an Expedition*. I remember how the tears rolled down my cheeks as I relived the anguish and pain that poured out of the canvas.

Eight years after my brother's death, my mom succumbed to cancer. She suffered with the disease for

three years, until, on the first of January in 1973, she joined my brother in a better place.

Should You Fire Your Boss?

Mental stress is huge when it comes to your health. We have managed to weave so much significance into our lives, and so much of it can have a stranglehold on our health today and in the future. Sometimes, this comes from your boss; if so, I recommend firing him. You might want to really look at this concept. If indeed you are working under unnecessary duress, your health now and in the future may depend on taking action, as scary as it may seem.

This may seem extreme, so what I recommend doing is writing down on a piece of paper two columns. Title the paper "In Five Years" or something like that. Write down in one column where you think you will be in five years if you stay employed where you are. In the other column, why not dream a little; write down what you would love to see happen in your life. What would be your ideal situation? After all, it is your life and you really can make it what you wish. Continue to write down thoughts for each of the two columns until you feel ready to

make a decision. If you decide its time to move on, then start to think about what you would really like to do with your life.

When I was about twenty-one years old, I got a job busting tires at Sears Automotive. That's right, here I am with a broken back, constantly in pain, and I took a very physical job. Well, I couldn't read and really had no other employable skills at that time, so I just dealt with the pain and kept going to the chiropractor to give me some sort of relief. I really didn't like the job and remember every year when my anniversary day came along, I would curse the fact that I was still there. Then one day, I was putting the largest size tire on this old guy's 1964 Lincoln Continental – those things were heavy – when the owner of the car spoke up. He told me that he was eighty-four years old and he could see that I had a bad back by the way I was moving and trying to lift those huge tires. He asked me how old I was and then said, "Son, you've got to get out of this business. If you don't, you will be crippled within a few years."

I went to my boss that day and told him I quit. The only thing was I didn't have another job lined up, so when he offered a sales job, I said okay. Now remember, I'd been a druggie for years and did not

feel comfortable talking to people, but I said, "Yes" anyway. For the next five years I kept that job. And I hated it. I dedicated nine years of my life to Sears Automotive. Every year when my hire date anniversary would come up, I'd ask myself why I was still there. I hate it here, I told myself.

Then one year I'd had it. I decided I hated the job so much that I might as well go back to school and get my chiropractic degree. I knew it would be very difficult, and I knew I had to confront not being able to read, but I decided I might as well go hate school for five years rather than hate working in the tire shop for the rest of my life. It was one of best decisions I ever made.

I know I said, "hate" a lot in this last paragraph, but it was true. I'm not a hateful person, I love life and I love people, but the situation was destroying my health, my attitude, and my back. So I quit –Yay! It may seem like an extreme idea, but life can be very short. It's time to enjoy every day like it is your last day on earth. So however this relates to you and your boss or your work, consider whether you are in the right place with a happy environment that can improve your health dramatically. After all, life should be fun and worth living, right?

How Do You Know Who is Making You Sick?

Sometimes your mental stress comes in the guise of a friend. Say goodbye and wish him well. Other times, this mental anguish comes from a family member, and this is a tough situation; the strain can come from your living situation or financial worries. Often times, we aren't even aware that we live in constant fear. Instead, it has become a lifestyle. Often times, we have gone on so long that we can't see the light at the end of the tunnel, and if we do, we are too afraid that it is a freight train and its coming fast. I wish I had a magic wand I could wave over your head to free you from this curse of the sentient mind. But rest assured, there is a magic wand and it is in you. Search for it. If you need help reach out, I'd love to talk with you!

Celebration of Life

Just yesterday, I attended a celebration of life for my dear friend, Don. He was my age and a very active, fun-loving adventurer. He was one of the best snow skiers I've ever known. Then, on December 23, 2019, he was skiing alone up in Lake Tahoe when he had a terrible accident that ended his life. His beautiful

twenty-three-year-old daughter spoke at his eulogy. She said something that came just at the right time for me. She said, "Choose your friends wisely in this short time on earth." She went on to say, "I now spend time with the people who mean the most to me." Then, Don's sister got up to talk about her fallen brother's life. She said something that Don had told her over and over throughout his life. This was so profound and was exactly what I needed to hear just at that moment; I think we all did. What she said was "You can always try one more time, but you can only quit once!" Wow, I wish my brother had heard that. When she repeated what Don would tell her, there was not a dry eye in the house. He was such an amazing man and this statement will follow me the rest of my life.

Okay, this may all seem so obvious, but are you really paying attention to your life? Who are those important people in your life right now? Where are they? When was the last time you spoke with them? Hugged them? Let them know you cared? If you feel compelled to put this book down and give them a call right now, please do!

Teaching from My Coach

I had a practice manager for ten years, named Dr. Jon Baker. He came at a perfect time in my life, and I owe so much to him for helping me find my way. We had a phone call every other Tuesday evening from six to six-thirty. So many times, Dr. Baker spoke to me about the situations I got myself into. My stress level was extreme, and many times I felt like giving up. Sometimes, I just wanted to crawl under a rock and disappear. However, I had three beautiful children to raise and a beautiful, loving wife. I had hundreds of patients who depended on me for strength and guidance. Dr. Baker had two messages for me that he repeated every two weeks for ten years. If I do my math, that's about 260 times. Dr. Baker had me write them down and read them every day. Sometimes, I would and other times, I'd be too stressed out to remember. Then, one day, I woke up worrying about something like, *What if the sun burned out*? I then came up with this revelation. Even though I'd been told it hundreds of times and read and repeated it to myself a million more, I came up with these two thoughts as if they were my own, and they were what Dr. Baker had drilled into this tiny pea-brain of mine:

1. Nothing has killed me yet!
2. 99.99 percent of the stuff I worry about never happens!

Wow, I finally got it. I knew, for myself, that this was true. I was still alive and nothing permanently devastating had happened to me. At that moment, my life changed forever.

There are many things and practices you can do to make this happen for you or for those you love. First off, just keep loving them, forgiving them, and forgiving yourself, and above all; decide to flourish and prosper and let them flourish and prosper.

Here are some of the exercises I've practiced to help me over the years. After all, to get good at any activity, you have to practice. Practice believing that you live a phenomenal life. Another thought Dr. Baker drilled into me over those ten years I worked with him was "What you think about, you talk about, what you talk about, you bring about!" Think wisely.

Here are some things that have helped me over the years:

Set Goals – Even If They Are Small Ones

Cut out pictures and stick them on your bathroom mirror. You can find anything you want on Google. Put up pictures of activities you have been unable to do because of your pain, build up in your mind that these can be done again.

I remember hearing a story of a Vietnam prisoner of war. He was kept in isolation for several years. He was kept in a cage that barely gave him room to sit or stand. He had one goal that he kept repeating over and again. He was a golfer, and he created a mental practice of playing a perfect round of golf. He would picture his favorite course and play each hole in his mind. He did this several times a day for all those years as a prisoner. And guess what, when he finally got out of the prison camp, his first goal was to play a round of golf. He had played that course so many times in his head that he did indeed play a perfect round. You are an amazingly powerful being. Don't be afraid of success. You can be, do, or have anything you desire.

Write Down A List of Positive Affirmations

Repeat them every morning. Spend five minutes, if even while in the shower, putting your future

there. This is so powerful. I had a coach who once said, “you will miss 100 percent of the baskets you never shoot.” As you work with these and repeat them over and over, they become more and more real. Pretty soon they are part of your nature and your makeup. Most actors, gymnasts, and acrobats visualize what they want to achieve. A good friend of mine has been a gymnast most of her life. She also has been an acrobat. She always wanted to do the flying trapeze. She thought about this a lot. She kept it so much in her desires that she finally found herself in Paris training with one of the best flying trapeze coaches in the world. When she finally got a chance to climb up the rope ladder to the flying trapeze, she had visualized the flight so much that she nailed it. This was not just a passing fancy, but a goal and desire, she knew it was going to happen, and it did.

Look to See Who Your Friends Are

Become aware of how the people around you are supportive, neutral, or destructive to your goals, creativity and emotions. Pay attention to how you feel when you are around them. You can ask questions of them and get a feel for if they support you

or not. You may know already. It's up to you, but if you value your life and your health, I'd say choose your friends wisely. Sometimes it best to quietly distance yourself from these people, other times it might be necessary to be a bit more overt in your separation of ways. This can be a delicate situation and sometimes ramifications will need to be considered. Please reach out to the email I provide if you have questions about how to handle this.

Make the Decision to Do the Physical and Chemical Practices I Outline

Basically inflammation is caused and sustained by what we put in our bodies. Whether it is food, drink, chemicals from work, or the garage etc., the sooner you learn which foods are good to add to your diet and which are bad and eliminate them from your diet, the better. I will elaborate on this concept in a later chapter, but for now, start paying attention to what you are putting in your body. Sugars, breads, any flours gluten free or not are not your friend. They are inflammatory. The sooner you can eliminate them the better. This includes sugary drinks and even sugar free drinks, juices and, of course, too much alcohol.

Use Dr. Baker's Thoughts to Help You Achieve A Wonderful Life

- Nothing's killed you yet
- 99.99% of the things you worry about will never happen
- What you think about, you talk about, what you talk about, you bring about

There is another friend who impacted my life with something he said every time I saw him. If you asked him how he was doing, he would always respond "*Great*, but getting better!" I always loved this and have adapted it for myself. I sometimes paraphrase it to "Awesome but getting Awesomer!" Try saying this for a week and see how you feel! Let me know!

One more gem from Dr Baker, He would say, "practice doesn't make perfect, perfect practice makes perfect." Find a purpose and go after it with everything you got!

CHAPTER 7:

Reducing Inflammation through the Cellular Healing Lifestyle

Okay, so you have heard me allude to how diet has something to do with your recovery from sciatica, and I'm not kidding. I have seen amazing changes in sciatic and other pain within a few days after clients changed their diets. Remember Dean? He was taking up to forty 800mg ibuprofen a week. As a construction worker, Dean was miserable, even though he wasn't doing as much of the physical work anymore. He was able to stop taking all forty ibuprofen, and this is how:

- He stopped eating all grains and all processed foods
- He started consuming six tablespoons of healthy oils a day
- He quit snacking between meals

Dean was able to achieve all of this, and he hadn't even started fasting yet, which we will get into in a bit.

I know this may sound crazy, and I must admit that I didn't believe it myself until I saw the same results over and over again, but this approach works. Now, everybody is different and each of us have our own cross to bear when it comes to food, but diet is as important to your recovery from sciatica as it is for you to enjoy the rest of your life.

Previously, I spoke about cellular inflammation and the damage caused by toxins like glyphosate and other man-made chemicals. Still, let's not forget about the intrusion of the opportunistic anaerobes, molds, and other viruses and bacteria. They are as deadly as death by a thousand lashes; they gang up on our bodies either by hitching a free ride or intending to kill us. These are all the subjects of this chapter.

You're Not Alone

At this point, I think it is important to discuss what happens at a cellular level. I'll keep it short, but if you are going to take control of your health, these are concepts you should understand. Understanding a bit about the cell wall will help you understand chronic inflammation.

If you put your hands in front of your face, palms facing each other but about an inch apart, this is kind of what the cell wall's construction looks like. Pretend one hand is the inside and the other hand the outside of the bi-lipid (two layers of oils) walls, meaning each of the walls are made out of lipids or oils and other substances. In the middle is a liquid (non-oil) substance, so basically we have lipid-liquid-lipid as the cell wall make-up. Intermingled along the wall are gates and channels that allow certain things to flow in and out of the cell. Certain vitamins, minerals, hormones as well as glucose and ketones travel through the cell wall through exact mechanisms. As long as the cell wall is healthy so is the cell and so are we.

Toxins from the environment and from our own cellular debris coming from things like energy production, not only clog up the cell walls and their

gates and channels but also organs like your liver and kidneys. This makes it very hard for your body's detoxification system to do its job.

This is an extant condition in our country; just look around at all the sick and unhealthy people. So suffice it to say, the more toxins we are exposed to, whether from our environment, our lifetimes, or passed down from Mom, the fuller our toxic load glass fills up and the more inflamed our bodies get. The longer the toxins stay in our bodies, the more likely it is that they turn on bad genes and cause cell mutation or genetic related disease to develop.

There are seventy-five to one hundred-thousand human cells making up our bodies. The one hundred trillion microbiomes in our intestines, as well as the unfathomable myriad which surround and encompass us, all depend on certain food stuffs for energy. Us humanoids have two choices when it comes to fuel: glucose or ketones.

Glucose is basically sugar, and this is the breakdown of every carbohydrate and protein we eat. Yes, take a moment here. Most people don't realize that protein is broken down and burned in our bodies as glucose, or sugar. Also, I can't tell you how many times I've mentioned to a patient to restrict their

carbohydrates, only to be told, "Oh, I didn't eat any carbohydrates today, I had a salad." It's okay, I totally understand; we have absolutely zero training in school about different types of food. I try to be supportive and encouraging as I explain to my clients that lettuce and broccoli are in fact carbohydrates and do burn as sugar. Also, it is rare that people understand that all protein, animal or plant-based, breaks down to and burns as glucose – or, you guessed it, sugar.

Toxins, including those opportunistic critters such as viruses, bacteria's, molds, and even parasites, are invading and attempting to disrupt our otherwise symbiotic relationship with our friendly microbiome which surround and intermingle with the cells of the human species. As Dr. Shane Morris, master biochemist and supplement formulator for the amazing Systemic Formulas company stated, "We are about seventy-five-trillion human cells but are covered or accompanied by at least ten times that in microorganisms, better known as the microbiome." He went on to say, "Nothing gets into our body without crossing through this massive complex called the microbiome." Without the microbiome to help us with environmental invaders, to help

us digest our food, or even to assist in the repair of our bodies, we would not have a chance.

Imagine the look on Dr. Jannsen's face when he first looked through his invention the microscope. All of a sudden, he saw something wiggling in that drop on the other side of the lens. At that moment in time, war was declared on the microscopic world. We've been spraying them, washing them, fumigating them, and if all else fails, burning them out. The silly thing is, they've been with us since the beginning. In fact, some of our own microbiome have traveled down through the centuries via Mom's birth canal, inoculating every generation since humans evolved on planet earth. You have strains of bacteria in you that existed as far back as we can imagine. If treated correctly, these guys can not only keep us healthy, but actually also slow down, and even help in, reversing the aging process.

A Rigged System Which Propagates Disease

If you look at the whole system set up to handle diabetes, a condition affecting 50 percent of Americans, we have too much sugar or glucose in our blood streams, and *all* treatment is designed

to keep the blood sugar levels within a safe (not healthy) range. Notice that these diabetes treatment plans make sure that patients eat six meals of processed, glucose-producing foods a day and are prescribed with enough medicine, like metformin or insulin, to push the glucose or sugar out of their bloodstreams fast enough so that it doesn't kill them. It is interesting how doctors have people with diabetes eat six small meals a day but say nothing about *what* people eat.

Here is the game; pretend you are the keeper of the floodgate, and if you open it too fast, it will kill the people below. This corresponds to the amount of glucose-producing foods that you eat. Now, let's say that I was the guy at the other end, dumping enough glucose out of your system fast enough to keep you alive (insulin or metformin). As long as we work together, things look pretty good, or do they? Where is all that glucose stored? This is the kicker – it is stored as fat. Our food consumption system is set up to feed us six glucose-filled meals a day to keep us filled up, but then we have insulin, produced by the body or man-made, to pull the glucose out of our bloodstreams as fast as it can, storing it as fat somewhere in the body. Where you might ask?

Again, it is stored as *fat*. The system is killing us. The longer this goes on, the fatter we get, until one day, it kills us.

Dr. Jason Fung is a well-known nephrologist; he spent his career working in the field of diabetes. He went to a good school, got a good education, and started treating diabetic patients in the conventional medical tradition. What he saw astounded him; he was not making his patients well but was only furthering them down a pathway to disease and certain death.

In an interview I did with him a couple of years ago, Dr. Fung spelled it out. Basically, what Dr. Fung said was, that by treating patients with medications such as insulin, he was able to get their blood sugar under control, but they also got fatter and sicker. He stated that by concentrating on only the blood glucose level and ignoring the rest of the patient's health, he felt that he was doing more harm than good.

Diabetes is the number one cause of kidney failure, preventable blindness, and limb amputation, and it increases your risk of cancer, heart disease, stroke, etc. Dr. Fung saw that even though the top hospitals in the country treated their patients the

same, no one was getting well, so he decided to relook at this epidemic.

At this point, Dr. Fung did two things. First, he stopped giving people the recipe for certain diabetic-related death, and second, he started investigating the alternative fuel source: ketones.

What is a Ketone Anyway?

We discussed glucose, but what is the other fuel anyway? Ever heard of a ketone? Quite honestly, based on the education of not only our fellow Americans, but also the lion's share of the medical profession, ketones are something people hear about in school, but they haven't seen one in years. By the way, if you do spot one, call the authorities immediately and stay as far away as possible. Of course, I'm joking, but not really.

What are ketones? Ketones are made in the liver by breaking down fat. Traditionally they are described as an alternative fuel source when you don't have enough sugar or glucose in your blood. Although this is true, the interpretation should be tweaked to say something like; Ketones are the "other fuel source." They are a clean burning alternative to the dirty, toxic burning of glucose which makes up

the standard American diet and has destroyed the health of several generations.

Ketones make an interesting story. In fact, in the 1920s, ketones were used to treat such conditions as seizures and other dietary-related conditions. Ketones were used quite readily and were successful, but the 1920s marked the dawn of the industrial age, and thus the sulfa drug revolution. Soon, profiteers had created a drug that controlled seizures. Even though ketones were basically free and not patentable, the drug was promoted, and soon after, the research papers and proponents of ketone use for seizures was lost in the woodwork. If you recall the power of the Rockefellers and their control over the expansion of petrochemicals, you can understand what happened to the simple and easy ketone approach to seizure treatment.

The FDA and the food cartels have brainwashed America into eating processed, sugar filled, vitamin deprived, and toxic foods, which predominately burn as glucose, and as a result American's have tremendous stores of ketones in the form of fat hanging on their bodies. The fact that converting your body to a ketone-burning machine, which decreases your dependency on glucose and stifles

your sugar cravings, can improve your health and decrease chronic inflammation seems to have been ignored by the powers that be.

There is a lot of misinformation out there and even misconceptions on how to safely partake in a ketogenic diet. And yes, there is a certain way to convert your body into a ketone burner, but this should be done correctly and also it should be understood that ketosis is something you want to move in and out of strategically. Remember, toxins of all kinds are stored in fat by your body's protective mechanism. Once safely stored in fat cells, the toxins aren't in circulation and are rendered harmless, temporarily. So an understanding of just how toxic you are is very important when you think about converting your body over. People often throw out the phrase, "I got the keto flu." This is a sign of burning fat too quickly or needing to actually get help professionally from a nutritionist, chiropractor, or health coach who understands how to help you detox or get into ketosis correctly. Caution should be had when attempting a ketogenic lifestyle.

What Can Fasting Do for You?

This brings me to the subject of this chapter, which includes the idea of fasting. Why fast anyway? Well, look down at your belly. Do you see all that stuff making your shirt bulge? That is a stored energy source that is not only healthy to burn, but it is also *free*. That is correct! You have enough stored energy on you to cut your food bill in half for at least six months; I just need to teach you how to tap into it. Don't worry, it is not that hard, and I will walk you through it.

In January 2019, Dr. Dan Pompa and a few of his Platinum doctors of which I am one, introduced to the world an amazing combination of dietary and health strategies designed to reduce chronic inflammation, restore cellular energy, eliminate brain fog, and reduce the chance of contracting any sort of age related disease. He introduced what I have now coined "The Cellular Healing Lifestyle." This includes intermittent fasting, the ketogenic diet, diet variation, cellular detoxification and ancient healing strategies. This multi-therapeutic approach is a game changer. I will roll out the process of how you can learn these techniques yourself in a link provided in the back of the book. If you have questions,

you will be able to contact me via my email, so that I can direct you appropriately.

Age Related Disease

We are now going to talk about that scary term "age-related disease." So, we have a couple factors here; one is the aging of the body and the other is the health of all the cell and organisms in, or of, the body. As an example of age-related conditions, let's consider a cut on the hand of a five year old, a forty year old, and an eighty year old; who would heal faster? Of course, the five year old would. Why? His body responds quicker, and his metabolism and survival index are higher.

When I talk about "age-related disease," I am talking about how the body is so overwhelmed with toxins that it can't find its way clear, so this is why I start with intermittent fasting. I want to *give your body a break*. Did you know that 65 percent of your body's energy is used up in digestive function? That's right – 65 percent of your calories go to digesting food, which is crazy. What if you stopped eating all the time? Could you let the body direct some of that saved energy to go do something important, like heal the broken or damaged bodily

functions? That is exactly what happens! In fact, one of the greatest chiropractors who ever lived was Dr. Reggie Gold. He always said this incredibly insightful phrase, "The body needs no help, just no interference." Wow – so the one principle behind fasting is allowing the body time to heal.

So, to heal your body, you need to start consuming more healthy fats, ketones, and eating less often by shortening your eating window. I will also walk you through the process of re-educating your body on how to burn this alternative "clean" fuel.

As these ketones burn clean, like a gas stove, they will actually help heal your brain from the toxic inflammatory build-up it has been exposed to via the "standard American diet." You want to burn ketones as your main fuel, not as an afterthought. This is the key to better health, and this is what Dean, Carol, Joe, and so many others did to help get the chronic inflammation out of their bodies. This was the start of a lifestyle that changed their lives forever.

Why Most Diets Fail

Now, let's take a look at why all diets fail. This is an easy concept to understand; nobody was ever

designed to have the same foods three times a day forever. This was a fabrication of the huge food corporations, like Kellogg's, who coined the "breakfast of champions" slogan when I was growing up. Back then, it was common knowledge what the "standard American breakfast" was – cereal (sugar), toast (sugar), and orange juice (sugar). Unfortunately, Mrs. Cleaver and Donna Reed believed their producers (you might be too young to get this point). T.V. promoted this concept, along with T.V. dinners, to a point that everybody wanted what was advertised. Where was the FDA for all this time? Now, two generations later, we are the most overweight country in the industrialized world and rate forty-ninth in the world for health. Thank you, Kellogg's and other mass conglomerates.

Let's take a walk down memory lane to our ancient ancestors. Here, we find a great lesson in our health potential. The concept of diet variation is not a new one, but it is not practiced, nor are its benefits understood at all. Our ancient families were forced to eat what was available. If it was a mammoth, first the family ate meat for a few weeks. Then, as winter approached, they ate the fat they had put away, stored roots, and the nuts. When

winter was over, our ancient families usually had nothing left. This was known as "starvation spring." They went without food until green things started to show up – first fruits and then later grains. They had to eat what was available, and this was actually a good thing because it kept the gut microbiome in check. So with the cellular healing lifestyle, I have incorporated strategies to help you use intermittent fasting and diet variation to mimic our ancestors' eating patterns. What I have seen is that our bodies love the challenge of variation and that the microbiome in our gut are challenged to a point where the unhealthy and harmful ones die off leaving healthier microbiome. All these bugs work well with our body's operating systems in a symbiotic relationship toward better survival.

Today, we have too many unhealthy strains of microbiome in our intestines. This is primarily due to the consumption of too many antibiotics. There are strains of antibiotics sprayed on our crops, put in the products we put on our bodies, and included in the chemicals we inject our animal-protein food sources with.

Thanks to modern science, we have scientists like Noble Prize winner Yoshinori Ohsumi and

scientists like Valter Longo who are proving that our bodies have the power to heal. Dr. Yoshinori Ohsumi defined autophagy in 2016 and created a greater understanding of how the body eats up the bad, weak, or cancerous cells in our bodies as a way of survival. What we know is that under times of stress, the body breaks down these older and weaker cells and allows for the byproducts of them to be recycled into new cells like stem cells. This is how the body regenerates itself.

The amazing thing is, we now have answers we never knew before. Terms like "autophagy" and "stem cell production" are becoming common words today, but there is a lot of confusion on how to do it and what to do. If not handled correctly, this can be a trap. Having a working understanding of fasting and the ketogenic diet along with ancient healing strategies, diet variation, and cellular detoxification will open the door for you to escape age-related disease, and actually turn back the biological clock (make you younger).

We also now know about things attached to our DNA that dictate our longevity. The cool thing is that recent science is proving that these things called "telomeres," which dictate our longevity,

can actually be bio-hacked to help us live longer and healthier lives! In a later chapter, we will discuss your health legacy and how to improve your chances for a healthy future. This is where you will learn to bio-hack your body.

There is so much information on the Internet these days that one would think that all they have to do is implement what they read. This may work for some people sometimes; however, I just want to recommend that you consider working with a health professional. Here are a couple reasons why; too often the data you read is incorrect and only partial at best, and often it lacks a complete understanding of the real purpose. Some people start these processes to lose weight or to gain energy, but so often because of things like toxic load build up or improper protein, carbohydrate or fat proportion the person fails, gets sick and gives up. These techniques when done correctly work like magic.

A great tool to get started is the Neuro Toxic Questionnaire. I offer this questionnaire on my website, and it will help you discover what your toxic load includes and to what extent, so you have a baseline to work from when you're ready to start working with a health professional.

CHAPTER 8:

True Cellular Detox

By this time, I believe you are getting the idea that your sciatica pain has a multifaceted etiology. I also hope that learning about the process of healing your body is giving you a few "ah-ha" moments.

When I finally made up my mind to get healthy and stop my back pain and sciatica, I was at the end of my rope. I had been living a life of quiet desperation and I needed a solution, come hell or high water, and I still had a dream of the high-water road. I finally realized that my attempts to handle my body had been mainly throwing more and more chemicals into it. As you'll recall, I had spent years putting everything from aspirin, to heavy pharmaceutical drugs, to street drugs into my body,

while constantly consuming pot and alcohol. I had a mouth load of silver fillings, which are 50 percent mercury, probably the deadliest heavy metal on the planet. I was addicted to sugar and hated eating anything green. By the time I was seventeen years old, I was diagnosed with a bleeding ulcer caused by my constant consumption of aspirin, usually followed by a shot or two of whisky or, in reality, a half bottle of Bombay Gin I stole from my dad. I was a mess. Lucky for me, I have a sister who cares about me. Thank you, Sudi!

The year was 1972, and natural healthcare was making a coming back. Big Pharma and petroleum industry had been flooding the United States with every kind of drug possible over the last many decades. Along with the media, owned by same corporations, the people in our country were duped or doped. One way or another, I was caught in the middle of it.

As I started to clean up my diet and quit taking the drugs, I noticed that I became more focused and able to think outside of the constant medications. When I met Dr. York on that fateful day, I was carried into his office, received my first chiropractic adjustment, and walked out on my own two feet. I made

a decision – I wanted to do what he did. I wanted to become a chiropractor.

However, as I mentioned earlier, there was a glitch, – I couldn't read. After being diagnosed with dyslexia in first grade, I was thrown down a destructive path, and breaking my back at a young age didn't help matters either. Well, this didn't stop me; I enrolled in Cabrillo College to try to get my pre-recs.

My first chemistry class proved fatal. There was a girl in my class named Jamie, who I liked. I sat next to her and hung out with her between classes, until one day I was so embarrassed that I dropped out of school. We had just taken our first quiz and received our test papers back from the teacher. I had received a very low D. The teacher asked us to pass the papers to our left and Jamie got mine as she passed hers away from me. That was when the teacher started berating us; he started telling us how pathetic we were, but then what he said sealed my fate. He said, "One of you was so stupid that you spelled 'acid' as 'asid.'" As I looked at my paper in Jamie's possession, I shriveled up into nothing. It took me another six years to attempt school again.

During that time, I discovered how toxic I was as I learned about mercury's toxicity. I even used to

play with mercury as a kid. I'd put mercury on dimes because it was so cool. My friends and I would go to our local five and dime store, called Merit Cycle and Toy, and buy games with liquid mercury in them and break them open to add to our collection. I remember putting the dime in my mouth; back then, nobody knew better. There was a grocery store called Star Grocery down the block, and they had this cool, liquid, plastic bubble toy. You'd put a glob of it on the end of a straw and blow these huge, liquid plastic bubbles, which was so cool. It was even cooler when you took the bubble and chewed it like bubble gum. I can't even imagine what kind of toxic petrochemicals I absorbed from that stuff!

On top of that, my grandmother owned a cotton ranch near Fresno. Every summer, I went to visit. One of the fun things we'd do was sit on the back of the tractor as my Uncle Bert drove up and down the rows of cotton. All my cousins and I had a wand, and we sprayed DDT, or some other toxic chemical, on the crops as we rolled along. Again, we didn't know any better. Sometimes, we'd just spray each other for fun. I developed asthma, while my dear cousin, Alberta, took the brunt of it and tragically died of lung cancer when she was way too young.

Man, I'd been exposed to so many toxins. It's amazing the toxins didn't cause permanent brain damage, but maybe they had! So began my road back to health. I was done being sick, tired of being in chronic pain, and sick of being labeled "stupid."

We've all lost loved ones. As you'll remember, my mother also died of cancer when she was fifty-six and I was seventeen. She developed ovarian cancer after the tragedy of losing my brother, and ultimately lost the long battle. As a kid, I remember the cloud of dust that surrounded my mother every day as she buffed talcum powder all over – and I mean all over her body. Today, we see TV commercials by attorneys touting statistics connecting ovarian cancer and the use of talcum powder, although this news came out a few decades too late for my mom.

Why did Alberta develop cancer? Why didn't I or my other cousins? What about my mom? What makes one person in the family so susceptible? Why could the rest of us do anything in the world and still be healthy as an ox?

Today, we have those answers and I can tell you one thing, "*size matters.*"

What do I mean by this? Science has come a long way, and with the unraveling and sequencing of

human DNA in the year 2000, a project which was conceived of in 1985 as the Human Genome Project, at University of California Santa Cruz, we can find the answers.

As the team of Human Genome scientists began to map out the 3.2 billion units of DNA strung together, which make up our genes, researchers discovered which gene did what, why, and how. This has allowed us to understand how certain genes get "tuned on" and cause bad things to happen. In the past decade, there was a huge movement to map out these different genes and find drugs to inhibit their "expression."

We have a long way to go, but now we know of many genes that cause things like colon cancer, breast cancer, Alzheimer's, certain types of arthritis, and the list goes on and on. There is even something called the MFTHR genetic defect, which has to do with vitamin B12 and B9 deficiencies and the body's ability to remove something called homocysteine from the blood. Homocysteine is a byproduct of energy production but is very inflammatory and can cause things like heart disease if not converted back to its parent metabolite with the help of the B vitamins mentioned above. With these discoveries,

pharmaceutical scientists were going crazy trying to be the first ones to find a drug to switch these genes "on" or "off."

For a while, this was cutting edge, but what we are currently seeing is that the body, and the life force in or around it, has an amazing ability to bypass these messed up pathways and find a new way around the defects. After all, these human bodies have stood the test of time, so far.

What makes one person susceptible to environmental toxins when another is completely oblivious to them? These people could walk through a minefield and still survive unscathed. Why is it that one twin sister, who grows up in the same house, goes to the same school, and eats the same food as her sister, will get sick or develop cancer, while her twin is as healthy as a horse?

This is where size comes in. Do you remember an actor named George Burns? He drank every day and smoked a boatload of cigars, yet he lived well into his hundreds. He was healthy, stubborn as a mule, and had all the mental capacities he needed to continue to entertain a nation, and then one day he just didn't wake up. Wow, that would be the way to go, right?

Size matters; it seems we were all assigned a glass when we came into this world, and this is our toxicity holding capacity glass. It could be a shot glass, a sixteen-ouncer, or an all-out bucket. We had no choice in its size nor how full it was when we were born. The glass was a luck of the draw. It's easy to see that our friend, George Burns, had a bucket.

As you'll remember from Dr. Bruce Lipton's cell membrane video (if you haven't watched it already, I am including the link here again: https://www.youtube.com/watch?v=5e8vB7AdcWI), Dr. Lipton says, plainly, the human cell when exposed to a toxic environment will immediately begin to die, but if that same cell is then put into a healthy environment it will immediately begin to flourish. Some of us were born with internal environments the size of a shot glass, some a sixteen-ouncer, and some of us were born with a bucket, like George. The point is that as long as your glass can contain the toxic load you are exposed to, as long as the detoxification pathway in your body is not clogged and is operating to keep your bloodstream, and thus your body, clean and healthy, and as long as you are lucky enough to avoid an overload of environmental toxins, you

might make it out alive. However, the lion's share of our country is not so lucky.

I want to take my hat off to the early adaptors in regenerative medicine, and the brave men and women who are defying the status quo and risking it all to go out on a limb and tell the truth. Thank you to people like Dr. Dan Pompa for taking on a band of hopeful doctors and healthcare providers and exposing us to a world where innate intelligence has rights, too.

In this world, we can unleash the body's ability to heal itself. We now have the tools. We have to tackle the toxicity in our body, and especially, and specifically, at a cellular level.

So, what is this about? How does this apply to me, you may ask? Here's how: true cellular detox. There are a few steps here, and all are doable. Once you understand how and why, I believe you will be the first on board.

Here is what we know; we have all been exposed to a truckload of toxins, without a doubt. The size of our toxin-filled glass will dictate if, and when, our body develops the diseases, age-related or not. Our individual genetic blueprint will have specific genes, and

if turned on, will dictate and unleash their expression, whether the disease is cancer, Alzheimer's, heart disease, cystic fibrosis, or who knows what else. Toxins in the way of chemicals, heavy metals, molds, viruses, bacteria, and their by-products, released as a result of hidden infections, damage first the cell walls, and then, just as the Mexican army swarmed the Alamo, these toxins enter the cell and even enter the cell wall of the mitochondria. Once the breaking point is met, we are doomed.

Did you know that we come into this world with our glass already loaded with toxins? That's right. According to Dr. Michael Skinner, an epidemiologist, who speaks about the fact that we are filled up with toxins that go back at least four generations. These toxins come to us through Mom's umbilical blood. So, if your great-great-grandmother had silver fillings (which are 50 percent mercury) and maybe worked in a smelting pot industry, all the toxins she received were passed on down the line. In fact, The Environmental Working Group, a non-profit American activist group, found 278 toxins in the umbilical cords of ten children who had not yet lived outside their mother's womb. These toxins contribute to the chronic inflammation in our

bodies and can augment the pain symptoms from conditions such as sciatica considerably.

So, our cups may runneth over before we even have a chance to step foot on this planet.

Of course, we live in the most toxic time in the history of the human race, so watch out. Our lifestyles and exposure to these toxic products continue to fill up our buckets; eventually, they spill over and we will go the way of the buffalo – near extinction.

In a *Cellular Healing TV* interview I did recently with Dr. Dan Pompa, episode 320 titled "New Hope for Sciatica," we discussed how as chiropractors who have both practiced for over thirty years. We recalled how years ago when a person receiving a chiropractic adjustment for something like sciatica they would respond relatively quickly depending on the physical component of cause. We both commented on the fact that today, chronic inflammation is responsible for increased physical pressure on the nerve to a point where chiropractic adjustments without also reducing or eliminating the toxic load and the ensuing inflammation often yields marginal results.

However, there is hope. We know how to empty our bucket, how to reduce our additional exposure

to more environmental toxins, how to repair the damage done to both the cell walls and mitochondrial cell walls (if we start soon enough), how to re-establish proper cell and organ-system communication and function, and how to restore proper communication through the powerful nervous and endocrine systems, and with a bit of determination and "luck," we can turn off the bad genes.

CHAPTER 9:

The Magic Light – How This New Stem Cell Machine Is a Game Changer

I'm about to tell you about the new stem cell machine that has changed my life and that of almost anyone it touches, but before I do, it is important to understand what it fixed and how I came upon this new tissue regenerative technology. It is straight out of Star Trek. Do you remember when Dr. McCoy, better known as "Bones," would wave his magic tricorder wand over any sick or injured crew member and they would immediately

recover? Well, if I hadn't experienced this myself, I would never have believed it. Let me explain.

Having been a chiropractor for the past thirty-plus years, I have put my body through hell. Making one-hundred-plus adjustments a day for thirty years physically demands my focus, energy, and willingness. Willingness has never been a problem due to my personal miracle adjustment performed over forty years ago. To that end, chiropractic never gets old. However, way back in the previous century, back when I was in fourth grade, I hurt my right shoulder, badly, trying to throw a softball as far as I could. My family had moved to a new town, my brother had recently died, and needless to say, I was not in what is now called "present time consciousness."

As anyone who moved to a different town growing up will tell you, it is important to work your way up the pecking order or be the one being pecked. So, throwing that softball must have torn a muscle or ligament of some sort, and my right shoulder bothered me ever since.

At twenty-one, I was arm wrestling a guy in the auto shop I worked at when he jumped the gun and my shoulder was reinjured. I remember the manager of the shop sent me to an orthopedist office for

evaluation. I felt intimidated by this doctor's arrogance, and without knowing I had a choice, I looked on in horror as he stuck a four-inch hypodermic needle full of cortisone into the ball and socket joint of my shoulder. I recall feeling sick like I needed to throw up as the whole four inches disappeared into my shoulder.

Years went by, and I routinely re-injured my shoulder. Many times, I had to drive, changing the gears of my model 2002 BMW with my left arm because I couldn't use my right. Eight months ago, I injured my shoulder so badly that I couldn't even lift it two inches away from my body. Believe me, I understand pain from many different angles. It's never the same, and every time, you can't help but wonder, "Is this the big one? Will I need surgery? Will that even work? I'm not going to go there; I have to get well."

This lasted for about three months. I even went to Mexico to get special platelet-rich plasma (PRP) injected into it. This helped a tiny bit, but not really. It's challenging to make every chiropractic adjustment you do for three months with only your left hand and not have anyone notice, although some people did.

Well, my cure – and I can call it that because it cured me – was to come in the wake of a dangerous and potentially fatal accident. My friend and colleague, Dr. Dan Pompa's son had a devastating injury when he attempted to jump off of a sixty-foot cliff into a lake. The thing was, he missed and landed feet-first on the rocks just above the water's surface. He shattered his ankles and fractured three vertebrae in his midthoracic spine. By Dr. Pompa's own testimony, his son should have died, or at least been paralyzed. As fate and faith would have it, this wasn't the case. In fact, because of Daniel Pompa Jr.'s training and resolve, he refused to be a victim. He knew that what his body needed was all the energy it could muster to heal. Against the advice from his team of doctors, Daniel decided to fast. He realized that the last thing he needed was inflammatory foods; after all, why waste 65 percent of his body's energy digesting food when it should be busy digesting and repairing damaged tissue?

Dr. Pompa and his son, Daniel, next embarked on the incredible journey to heal Daniel's back. No holds were barred in order to help Daniel's body heal. Dr. Pompa had the availability of many alternative machines and therapies to assist in the healing. One

of the machines was a TRT, or Stem Cell Machine. It has been named the “Miracle Machine” by many of my patients and the “Stem Cell Machine” by the physicians on the TV show *The Doctors*. Suffice it to say, Daniel was not only walking, but also traveling to Europe within four weeks of the injury. The surgeons were astounded, and the rest of us came away with an even stronger belief in the idea that the body can heal itself.

I’ve been a colleague of Dr. Pompa’s for over four years, and along with about forty other dedicated regenerative enthusiasts, we partake in almost any experiment or study Dr. Pompa throws our way. What we saw early on after Daniel’s injury was treated, was that this new technology was a miracle and a testimony to life’s innate ability to heal itself. This was my introduction to tissue regenerative technology, or the TRT machine.

When I saw the results in just one treatment on Daniel, I asked Dr. Pompa where I could find one. He introduced me to a guy named Dr. Matt DiDuro in Atlanta, Georgia. I was dismayed to find out there weren’t more than fifty of these machines in existence in the United States. I desperately asked Dr. DiDuro to find me the closet one, and he finally

located the only one in Northern California at the time. I told him I was willing to drive hours to find it, and I did.

In my eyes, what happened next was a true miracle. Now, I did have an idea of what to expect having talked to Dr. Matt and seeing a video of Dr. Pompa performing treatment on his son's back. But nothing could have prepared me for what I experienced on my first treatment.

Now, as you know, I've been in practice for a long time and have tried almost every new or ancient modality ever conceived of. This TRT, Stem Cell, or Soft Wave machine, whatever you want to call it, blew me away. Not only did it give me immediate relief, but it also seemed to know where the problem was. The machine found the problem in the most unexpected of places. The machine has been described as being able to diagnose and then treat the lesion or chronic injury within ten minutes, and it did. The wand of the machine is filled with water. There is a filament in it that snaps light at a certain frequency, which can detect damaged verses healthy tissue. Since there is really nothing to compare it to in existence, you really have to experience it yourself. The ten-minute treatment I received with

that machine resulted in an immediate 40 percent decrease in pain and a 40 percent improvement in range of motion in my shoulder. For the first time since fourth grade, I had hope that I might finally recover.

The following week, I rescheduled my patients and made the drive back to the magic machine. That time, I walked away 80 percent better. That was it, I bought one, and it ain't cheap, but the best things in life aren't. This was the best decision I've ever made regarding my patients and my practice. Since purchasing my Stem Cell machine in September 2019, I have had success with a plethora of conditions, from TMJ (temporal mandibular joint disorders), diabetic neuropathy, shoulder pain, elbow pain, hand pain, knee pain and dysfunction, back pain, and even sciatica. In fact I now use it in almost all my protocols. Its use has not only improved outcome but also shortened the necessary length of care, markedly.

I was the first one of Dr. Pompa's group to buy a Stem Cell machine, and since that date four months ago, almost twenty of the other doctors in the group jumped on board. The doctors and health professionals of Health Centers of the Future are

definitely early adaptors, and we now have an army of TRT-equipped Health Centers of the Future doctors out there changing the world. This is the caliber of doctor involved in HCF; we pull no punches when it comes to helping our clients and patients. In addition, we stand united to help change healthcare in this country.

Now, some of my best friends – our team of Health Centers of the Future clinicians – meet around the world to explore the newest, and often controversial and ground-breaking, treatments and technologies so that we can bring them to you.

What Is TRT and What Does It Do?

First, let me say the recent introduction of this machine into the US leaves it little known by the major medical complex, and it will no doubt be a while until its amazing results catch on. It goes by several names – TRT, Soft Wave, "The Stem Cell Machine," or the Shock Wave. I believe time will help establish its "handle." But, for now, we will call it the TRT machine to keep it easier.

Tissue regenerative technology is considered a shock wave therapy. The best way for me to describe how the mechanism of TRT machine works

is such. The TRT machine creates shock waves. These shockwaves bypass healthy cells having no effect on them but, evidenced by my own experience, when the shockwaves pass over damaged tissue, they will mimic the previous injury, sending a signal to the brain that there is a "new" injury. This triggers the brain to set dormant stem cells, which reside in your bones, into motion to go fix the injury. There is also evidence that this creates angiogenesis, or new blood vessel growth, at the site of application. This is cool because it means that there will be more nutrition available as well as a more efficient cleansing of the area because of blood circulation.

For a more in-depth view of how shockwaves from TRT promote tissue regeneration, I highly recommend TRTLLC's Shockwave Summary article that breaks down this process in more detail.

What about Stem Cell Injections? Pros and Cons

Stem cell therapy is getting a lot of press these days, and I wanted to take a minute to discuss this and some precautions to be aware of. Not all stem cells are the same; there are several different ways to collect them. The industry is still in its infancy and

there is a lot of false or unverified claims out there. However, there are many patients who have had great successes with the various procedures.

I think the important thing is to know how to do your research and what questions to ask, and I will give you a little bit of information on this. This information is not intended to be a treatise on the subject of stem cells, but to at least broach the subject to bring some questions and thoughts to the forefront.

There was a period of time when the practitioner would extract your own stem cells from the fat cells in your belly or from the bone marrow. It has been said that both together would be good, but depending on your age, you are getting less healthy cells. The older you get, the less successful the procedure.

Today, the industry is looking to umbilical stem cells harvested from donor mothers. These should be highly regulated, and the blood should be scanned for many things. I know that Dr. Raphael Gonzales's World Stem Cells Clinic in Cancun, Mexico has an extensive and rigorous screening process to ensure that the stem cell donors are free of issues.

In speaking with Dr. Gonzales, I am aware of the fact that over 75 percent of the cords are rejected

for any number of reasons. A few are rejected when screened because several viruses can be detected. These can be Epstein-Barr virus (EBV), cytomegalovirus (CMV), chronic infection, and particularly any genetic defect, to name a few.

Another thing that Dr. Gonzales' clinic does, which is actually not allowed in the United States, is the replication, or multiplication, of the stem cell harvest. The cool aspect about this is that when you are infused with the stem cells you end up with a more plentiful dose and you know that you are getting a thoroughly culled and safe dosage.

There is no real standard for stem cells in the United States yet, and it is still the wild frontier. For instance, the fact that there may be a few live cells in a culture allows the clinic to call them "live." There are a multitude of practitioners jumping on the bandwagon trying to get a piece of the action. I would be careful about trusting sources of stem cells at this point. There is no guarantee of the quality or quantity of stem cells available in your dosage yet.

The beauty of going outside the United States is that the restrictions don't apply, and if you go to a known clinic, like Dr. Gonzales' World Stem Cell

Clinic in Cancun, not only can you feel comfortable with the quality of the product, but you can also enjoy the beautiful location as well.

Nevertheless, please do your own research and feel free to reach out if you have questions. Feel free to contact me if you would like an introduction to Dr Gonzales' clinic.

Extra-Corporeal Stem Cell Recruitment

One of the cool things about the tissue regenerative technology machines is that it operates *extra-corporeal*, which means that it is non-invasive. The sound wave machine operates from outside the body, so one of the many great things about this machine is that it recruits your own stem cells to the site of application. It also induces new blood vessel growth, which is amazing for diabetics, as patients' extremities are challenged by clogged capillaries. Chronic inflammation is reduced dramatically, and acute inflammation is held at bay.

The amount of success that my colleagues and I have with the TRT machine is unprecedented, and the success stories are almost unbelievable. You actually almost have to be there to see the results. In the back of this book, you will find links to many

different doctors' sites where you can find story after story of pain relief, increased mobility, improved function, and more from the TRT miracle machine. For direct contact with the source, go to TRTLLC.COM. You will find up-to-date research and the many FDA approved usages for the machine.

When you are ready, I will help you find a TRT owner as close to you as possible.

To recap, the shock wave machine has been evidenced to have these effects.

1. Reduce cell death (Apoptosis)
2. Reduce inflammation
3. Induce sprouting of new blood vessels (angiogenesis)
4. Induce stem cell recruit, both exogenous (not yours) and within your body
5. Improve erectile dysfunction
6. Improve wound healing
7. Pain reduction
8. Induce neuronal regeneration

There are currently several studies underway to further understand usages for this amazing technology. Not all usages above are done in my office;

however, referrals to the appropriate provider can be arranged for those interested in such.

I have been the proud owner of a tissue regenerative technology "Stem Cell Machine" since September 2019, and the number of miracles it has produced in my office is astounding. Sciatic pain has been diminished to zero often times by the first treatment. Other times, depending on the multifaceted factors causing the problem, healing may take longer. Three to five treatments per area is what is recommended. If we don't get results by then, we consider missing factors. There are the three big ones:

1. Heavy metals
2. Molds
3. Hidden infections.

Not to exclude physical impingement from misaligned vertebra or muscle contraction along the nerve track. I will discuss how these can hamper your progress and what steps to take in a later chapter.

CHAPTER 10:

Developing Your Health Legacy

"The body needs no help; it just needs no interference."
—Reggie Gold.

Now that you're at this chapter, I hope you see what your future health and life could be like. You may have a new understanding of your previous thought and operating systems regarding your health, what you put in your body, and what you do when you have any symptoms (pain, loss of energy, trouble sleeping). You may also have a better understanding of who actually influenced your ideas about what health is and how to "fix" it when

it starts to fail. Television, newspapers, magazines, as well as the local doc-in-the-box have taken their toll. Worry not, there is yet hope!

You've probably changed the way you eat and have started to get some more energy back. Just by changing what you put in your body alone will change your life. So many of my patients announce that their sciatica, back pain, leg pain, headaches, and cravings diminish after the first couple of weeks of cleaning up their diets.

You might be beginning to understand that sciatica, as well as most disease, is a multifaceted condition. There is no doubt that the physical component needs to be addressed, and I have some exciting news for you coming up in the next chapter. Please understand that we are shooting for a complete reversal of this condition, so it is important that we get to the bottom of your condition.

These are some of the results my patients have reported around the second or third week of simply changing what they put in their mouths:

- Weight loss
- Pain relief both acute and chronic
- Increase in energy

- Loss of brain fog
- Younger looking (and people comment on this)

Some other results I see as patients continue to implement these techniques are:

- Stronger immune system
- Reduction in chronic disease syndromes
- Lower blood pressure lower
- Cholesterol and triglycerides in check
- Reduced need for certain medications (I had several diabetic patients whose medical doctors reduce their Metformin and other insulin-like drugs)
- No need for any pain killers (Dean no longer took forty ibuprofen a week, Trisha stopped taking twenty-one ibuprofen)

It is exciting to watch people's lives change right before my eyes as they begin to embrace their health in a new light! The very cool part is that this is not very hard to do. In fact, all these patients did at this point was as simple as cutting out grains, breads, and sugars and consuming healthy fats such as avocado oil, olive oil, coconut oil while cutting out the

bad polyunsaturated oils we've been taught to eat. They have counted how many times they actually put some sort of food in their mouths and then cut out the snacks, consuming three keto friendly meals a day. With these simple steps, they have started to embrace this new anti-inflammation lifestyle:

Generally, by this time, patients have made several decisions regarding their health. Often times, they are a bit pissed off that nobody showed them how to do this before, and other times they are incredibly happy, but almost all are blown away by what happened to them over the years, and they are amazed at the ability of the body to heal itself. They typically all realize that the "age related disease" thing can pass them by and that they can actually start to feel younger.

There becomes a general understanding that this new way of looking at your health – this new responsibility – brings with it not only a new way of living, but also an opportunity to help others. I have had so many of my patients tell me that they have a son, sister, mother, or cousin somewhere around the country, or the world, in need of this information. They ask me to try to help them. Many patients have brought their friends and family members into this

new way of life. As I spread this information and the techniques to reduce inflammation, chronic or acute, and as we start to scrutinize and restrict what we put in our bodies, and in the bodies of those we love and care for, we begin our health legacy.

Why would we want to create a health legacy anyway? Health is a private thing, isn't it? Aren't the HIPPA laws there to keep our health secrets hidden?

A good friend of mine and an amazing healer, Dr. Mindy Pelz, made a great statement the other day, saying, "Isn't it crazy how we are involved in groups in so many areas of our lives? Those of us who are religious hang with like-minded people. If we are in a profession, we have associations; we have a family unit, and in college we are in fraternities or sororities, but when it comes to our health, we are very private!" Wow, what an observation, and it is so true.

How did this come about and why? In the times of our ancestors, and even in more remote civilizations and cultures on the planet today, when a member of the community becomes ill or injured, the community is there to support them. Who has gained anything by making us feel ashamed, belittled, handicapped, or hopeless when it comes to our health conditions? Here is a thought, maybe if you

told your friends or family members what you were being prescribed or about what you've been indoctrinated with by the merchants of Big Pharma, you might decide to look up and see that there is more to health than meets the eye. What if everybody on this planet believed in the fact that our innate intelligence, given a chance and free of toxic overloads, could heal our bodies?

Remember Dr. Reggie Gold,, DC's bold statement, "The body needs no help, just no interference"? If you feel that it is time to allow your body to heal itself, then you are in the right place. Dr. Pompa has paved the road and solidified the processes and techniques. He also keeps us current on all the new developments out in the wonderful world of regenerative medicine. The group of doctors I am so happy to be part of are constantly studying, investigating, and putting to practice the latest breaking science available.

Dr. Pompa's statement, "fix the cell to get well." says it best. After all, life begins and ends in the cell. What Dr. Pompa taught us are the five steps to restore our cellular energy in order to allow our bodies to heal, so we can get our health back. He constructed the five Rs, which actually take your body

through the steps necessary to accomplish just that. His five Rs roadmap to achieve optimum health are:

1. **Remove the sources of toxins in our life**: Uncover where in your life and environment toxins are located, whether they're under your kitchen cabinet, the garage, your detergent, soaps, in your medicine cabinet, deodorants, or make-up. Once you go through your house and pull all the products out, read the labels and warnings. There is an app called "Think Dirty," which you can download on your phone. This is cool because you can scan the bar code with your phone and actually find out what is in the product. The app scores or rates the chemicals from one to ten, with ten being bad and one being good. You can make decisions on what to keep and what to send to the toxic waste dump.
2. **Regenerate the cell membrane or wall**: This is all about learning what good oils to eat and which ones not to eat, finding out what foods to avoid because they cause inflammation or damage to your cell walls, as well as what causes toxic waste inside the cells as foods are burned for fuel. A healthy cell wall consists of

healthy oils, proteins and other substances. At least 35 percent of the cell wall is made up of good omega-6 fatty acids. Making sure you are eating the right organic oils such as coconut oil, avocado oil, ghee, or olive oils will start you on the right path as you learn how to eat organic foods.

3. **Restore cellular energy**: As you do steps one and two above, begin to introduce certain vitamins and foods that have the correct proportion of nutrients in them to feed the mitochondria and other cellular organelles (great word, meaning little mechanism in the cells that assist in the production of life,). Today we know that certain nutrients enhance the power of the cell. There are certain companies, which I recommend for their purity and consistency. Systemic Formulas is my favorite. It is important in this step to get some help understanding what your particular body needs. You can waste a lot of money buying things your body can't absorb or doesn't need.
4. **Reduce inflammation**: Depending on an individual's toxic load and health index, including

any "disease" processes going or autoimmune issues (where the body is actually attacking itself), a recipe for success can be created. Once you have achieved steps one through three above, the body will start to function healthier. It may take a bit of time, but it is worth the effort.

5. **Reestablish methylation (energy production)**: Now you have a body that has cells and an internal environment that is so clean that the cell powerplant burns efficiently on ketones so that copious amounts of dirty burning glucose and insulin are not needed to run the body. The cells have adapted and become able to burn "the other fuel," ketones, as well as glucose. It's like having a smart car that can burn gas or electricity as needed to be as efficient as possible. Have you seen a car driving down the road with blue smoke pouring out of it? This is how a lot of our bodies burn fuel. If you look in the mirror and you don't like what you see or feel that you are burning fuel like that car I just described, just know that you have a choice; I have a path that you can follow.

These steps will help remove the toxins from your internal environment, allowing your body to turn on good genes and turn off bad genes. By detoxifying the cell and getting the membrane healthy, your body will be able to recognize and utilize hormones without the need for mass quantities of Big Pharma's concoctions, which has actually been furthering the demise of America's health, driving us close to the worst health index in the industrialized world. Is it time to take back your health?

Summary

Now it is more important than ever that you, me, and everyone we know thinks about and creates our own health legacies. Hopefully we have all realized by now that the wrong people have had too strong of an influence regarding our health. You probably understand that your sciatica or any other condition you may have is multifaceted and may require the same type of treatment to get well. You have learned about techniques to reduce inflammation by changing what you eat. And you will likely be able to wean yourself off the pain meds, which have only made things worse over time. You also learned that cutting out inflammatory foods such as grains

and sugars can reduce inflammation. Finally, you've learned that to consume three keto friendly meals a day will reestablish a healthy cell wall.

Once you have made a decision to take control of and change your health, then you will change your life. You are starting to understand that your body has the ability to heal itself as long as you get the interference out of the way and allow your own body's immune system to do what it was designed for. Then, by implementing Dr. Pompa's 5 Rs your body can start to truly heal and you will start to fix and heal your body on a cellular level.

Remember, Sciatica is a multifaceted condition. To truly remedy yourself from this issue, your willingness to do something different is necessary.

CHAPTER 11:

Planes, Trains, and Automobiles

I can't tell you how many patients spend hours in the hot tub having the blower pound their point of pain. This feels good for a while but causes so much inflammation in the area that people often crawl away with debilitating pain. Sometimes massage therapists can help, but too often they dig into the point of pain, which feels good at the time, but again, has huge ramifications.

So, here is my point – there is no real quick fix. Sure, you may get relief through many different modes of treatment, and by all means go for it, as long as the provider knows what they are doing. But as far as a magic bullet? Forget it.

I've been on probably every side of sciatica, both as a practitioner and as a patient. In fact, when I was in my seventh quarter of chiropractic school, I worked construction to help pay my tuition. One job required me to use a jackhammer to knock out a foundation. The position I had to get into to do this was ridiculous. It was such a bad angle that I completely blew my back out – again. I could barely walk. I was in so much pain and at such an antalgic position (leaning severely off to the left), that it took me ten painful minutes to walk to my next class. I had two choices: drop out of school for a quarter and lose all of my study buddies (which was important since I still didn't have the reading thing down), or just suffer on through. So I decided it best to suffer.

I went to almost every single chiropractic teacher on campus and no one – I mean, *no one* – would adjust me. I was in so much pain and so unable to move that I thought it was finally over. However, what shocked me most was that there wasn't a single chiropractor teacher who would touch me for "liability reasons." I guess that is why teachers teach, right?

In desperation, I went into the field and found a chiropractor who was not afraid to treat me named

Dr. Brian Coyle. This guy had me free of pain and up and walking in one week – amazing. What this taught me was that even in chiropractic school, the medical influence was encroaching. More importantly, the power that made the body could heal the body. It just needed the ability to communicate and get rid of the nerve interference.

My point here is, great, get out of pain any way you can (without becoming a drug addict or drinking yourself to death), but realize that the only way to a pain-free and incredibly optimistic future is to go "up-stream" to the actual causes of your health condition and handle it on all levels so that your twilight years can be yours to enjoy and remember.

When a new patient walks, crawls, or is carried into my office, or any doctor's office for that matter, they usually want four things. They want to get in and out quickly, to get out of pain, to avoid spending any money, and to never see that doctor again – who can blame them? Our healthcare system has become a sickness-care system. Big Pharma has rigged it so that all we do is manage disease and its symptoms. The citizens of this country are considered "consumers" to the pharmaceutical companies, and why in the hell would you want to limit or cut

down your client base? It would be suicide for the industry if people actually started to get well.

When I see a new patient for any kind of pain-related problem, such as neck pain, lower back pain, sciatica, shoulder, wrist, hand or leg pain, there is a common question they almost all ask, "What stretch or exercise can I do to help get rid of this pain?" My answer is usually close to, "Nothing yet!" Why? There are several reasons. Typically, the patients have already tried everything and inflamed the condition worse than it originally was. Other times, patients continue to work out, stretch, get bodywork, or have their kids walk on their back while on one, or several, pain meds or anti-inflammatories, making things worse.

Remember, pain (or other symptoms) is there to let you know something is wrong. When you mask the pain or symptom with drugs and either continue on with life as if nothing is wrong or try some new exercise or drink your neighbor's favorite concoction, you are blunting your body's awareness systems, which can have bad results.

As a kid, I remember the first time I got Novocain at the dentist. It was such a weird sensation, and I noticed that it didn't hurt to bite the inside of my

cheek – yikes. So, I actually chewed a hole in my cheek. Man, when that Novocain wore off, boy, was I in pain. My cheek took a week to heal. My point here is that covering up symptoms with pain meds or other drugs can be dangerous.

Take Dean, for instance. He was consuming forty 800mg of ibuprofen a week for several years to cover up his pain so he could continue to work. By doing this, Dean continued to wear out the spinal discs in his back, causing severe degenerative arthritis, but he was also doing an untold amount of damage to not only his liver and kidneys, but also to the arterial walls of his blood vessels. Recent studies are proving that constant consumption of NSAIDs can be a causative factor in Alzheimer's disease. In fact, almost all drugs from antacids to prednisone are being linked to Alzheimer's.

Again, here is my point – there is no shortcut to better health; it has to be a lifestyle change. Sure, we can help you get pain relief, and chiropractors, acupuncturists, and medical professionals all have their ways of doing this, but if you are at a point where you see the writing on the wall, and when you are coming to grips with the fact that your biological clock is running low, or you have a dream to live

into your twilight years enjoying the golden years, playing with your grandkids and remembering their names, then a lifestyle change is for you.

My hope is that you make the change before it is too late, and before you fall into the grips of irreversible chronic disease.

CHAPTER 12:

The Long and Winding Road

By going through the pages of this book, I hope that you had a few realizations; I surely had them while writing it. Perhaps you have seen improvement in your pain level, your energy, and your outlook on life already. My goal is for you to make it all the way to the goal line. The road can be bumpy and booby-trapped, but with a little help from your friends, you can make it.

So, now it's time to make a decision. You may have started reading this book to finally figure out how to handle your sciatic pain. In the process, you've no doubt found that there is more to it than a "pinched nerve." Even if your condition was a bit

less complicated, and I hope it was, there is a lot of room to improve your overall health.

There is an old blues song by the late Albert King, entitled "If the Washing Don't Get You, the Rinsing Will." Albert was teaching us that life is filled with pitfalls and sometimes we can't help the cards we are dealt. I used to play this song in my younger years and actually went into agreement with it. It seemed like no matter what happened, the other foot still had to drop. I just couldn't seem to get out of my own way. There were always obstacles in the way. Many were visible, and the others were imaginary, but no matter what their makeup was, I just kept running into them, one after another. Then, that fateful night came when my heart almost stopped, and I truly felt my life was over. That was the turning point – there was no going back. And as I moved forward with a good understanding of how the body works and what heals it, I found hope and got the help I needed to get well. Regardless, our health is our own responsibility; nobody cares as much about your health and well-being as you.

There will be a lot of difficulties and setbacks on your journey to an amazingly healthy, productive and fulfilling life. To make this road easier for you,

I have set up courses and classes to help. I even have online meetings that you can join and participate in.

Life is too short to live it in pain or ill-health. I recommend not going it alone. We have seen amazing improvements with the recent discoveries and breakthroughs in natural science. Whether you decide to go it alone or allow us to help, I thank you for your time. Please let others know about this book so that they may find help as well.

Now, let the healing begin!

First Off, "Get me out of pain!"

There are certain things to help you right away. Getting a thorough spinal exam by a qualified corrective care chiropractor can give us the lowdown on what is actually going on at a spinal level; we need this info. Most orthopedists, neurosurgeons, and physiatrists look for something to drug, burn, or cut. No offense to them – they are only doing what they've been taught – but the statistics are not in their favor.

Once we know what the scoop is in regard to spinal degeneration – old injuries resulting in things like spinal misalignments, "subluxations," healed compression fractures, or boney abnormalities

(genetic or acquired) and the general state of your spinal column – we can proceed to get you relief. Once you get the results of your examination and full body spinal x-rays, if you would like me to review them, please feel free to contact me.

After this evaluation, we can determine if you are a candidate for the "Miracle Machine," better known as the "Stem Cell Machine," utilizing tissue regenerative technology. If so, we will find the closest practitioner to you. At the time I am writing this, there are less than eighty TRT machines in private practice in the United States, so there is a chance that you will need to set aside some time for a journey, but it will be worth it.

I currently have people driving over three to four hours each way to receive a TRT treatment in my office. The results are amazing. As this machine gets more and more exposure, I believe I will need to purchase another just to keep up with the demand. Hopefully, more practitioners will find out about it. A couple obstacles stand in the way of popularizing these machines; first, most doctors are often too busy handling emergencies to keep their eyes open for these miracle machines. Secondly, the machines are extremely expensive. In fact, if the TRT machine

hadn't fixed my shoulder in two visits, there would have been no way I would have considered buying one. After seeing the results, I had no choice.

What we find is that the worse the condition, the better the results with the TRT machine. At any rate, I found that correcting the spinal condition can be achieved with a lot less chiropractic care. The combination of TRT and chiropractic to correct the underlying cause is often cut in half. This is amazing but let me define "correction." This does not get you a perfect spine, but it gets you the spine you brought in working as best as possible. Believe me, your body does have the ability to heal. The more physical, chemical, and mental interference we remove, the better the results.

If the TRT machine is not in your reach, and I hope it is, there are still plenty of things to do to turn your health around, but remember, this is just the beginning. If you want to heal and live a long and vibrant life, then it is important to handle the rest of your body's contributing issues.

When it Comes to Your Health, Remember T.E.A.M.

You will recall that my good friend Dr. Mindy Pelz, made a statement that completely resonated with me. She said, "It's funny how people love to hang out and do things in groups. Whether through religion, sports, clubs, or just groups of friends, we are social animals, but when it comes to our health, we keep it private." I know I mentioned this before, but I think it is important to look at this now. I love the acronym T.E.A.M. (together we all achieve more), and I believe that if we apply this to our individual healthcare we could, and would, change the health of our group, then our community, and then the health of our nation.

Einstein said something like, "The definition of insanity is doing the same thing over and over again, but expecting different results," and you can relate this to your journey with sciatica.

This is why I am so excited to bring this new multi-therapeutic approach to sciatica to the forefront. Also, I'm here to tell you that my experience is, working with groups of patients to improve their health has not only been fun but has proven to be far superior in effectiveness than working with

individuals. We are on the precipice of a major shift in the way Americans and perhaps the world views health care. The take home message is, "if it's to be it's up to me." This has never been more clear than today. We have no "Magic Pill" to fix our health.

So, if you are serious about getting your health back, you have a couple choices that may work:

1. Do nothing and continue down the road you are on.
2. Keep to yourself and try to improve, and maybe you can.
3. Join up with an amazing group of people excited about their health today and into the future.

Personally, I like the last one; selfishly, I like this one because it is so fun getting to know people and watching them win in life again. And, we can share the latest breakthroughs in health and regenerative medicine the moment they appear in the literature.

Becoming a "Health Rebel" against the Old Health Paradigm

I started a private Facebook group called "Health Rebels" about a year and a half ago with the purpose of helping individuals find a better way to live a healthy and prosperous life. We as a group have embraced many health challenges by looking at how we can help the innate power within our own bodies to flourish. We have people from across the country contributing to our cause. I highly recommend that if you are on Facebook to join this group. I believe we will all rise up together to a new understanding of how our body heals and what we can do to help ensure it does.

Just so you know, you don't have to live in Santa Cruz by the beach to be a part of our group. We have some amazing online courses that include live Zoom meetings where we meet face-to-face as a group and debug any issues. I also have private counseling and coaching for more complicated cases if that is your desire or sounds more appealing to you.

Additionally, being a Health Centers of the Future doctor, I am affiliated with over forty practitioners across the country and have a direct line to Dr. Dan Pompa. We meet weekly to continue our exposure to

the latest breakthroughs, and these breakthroughs are happening at lightning speed. More importantly, we run difficult cases through the group. This last thing is invaluable.

Many practitioners are busy and confined to their practices, working tirelessly to keep up with their patient load. God bless them, but often times they work alone and don't have time to keep up with the current breakthroughs. I can tell you one thing – what was true yesterday in health is old news today. It takes a team of early adaptors to bring the latest information into our offices to benefit the lives of our patients.

I want to address cost right off the bat. Health does not have to cost an arm and a leg, no pun intended here, but considering the costs of not fixing your failing health and continuing down the bumpy road to old age, like so many of our friends and family do. It can be far more costly in time, disease, pain, loss of mindfulness, finances, and perhaps most importantly, happiness.

If you are interested in utilizing my program independently, that is not a problem. I have set up some amazing online courses, which will walk you through the process of turning back your biological

clock. You can go to www.mccollumwellness.com for more information on various classes, which I will list below as well.

Cellular Healing Lifestyle Workshop

This is a seven-week intermittent fasting ketogenic online course (or in-house for locals) that walks you through everything you need to do to bio-hack your body and start healing, as well as turn back the biological clock.

Science has shown that the one way to reverse the aging process and to help clean up the inflammation in your body is by fasting. There are different kinds of fasting. Intermittent fasting is a biggie these days. By fasting, we know you will burn up easy to burn fuels in your body. This could be old, weak cells that get broken down through a process called autophagy or self-eating. Under times of stress, and especially when the food sources are scarce, the body looks for and burns its more useless cells to sustain life. This was discovered and explained by Dr. Yoshinori Ohsumi, winner of the 2016 Nobel Prize for medicine and physiology. He discovered that the body, under times of stress (or fasting) does not burn the good, healthy muscle

but the weaker and less productive cells and other tissues in the body.

The Keto diet has gotten a lot of press these days because ketones, which are broken down when fat burns, burns clean, kind of like a gas stove. Any other fuel, like protein and carbohydrates, burn dirty, like a wood burning fireplace filled up with wet, smoky pine. It burns, but it is toxic. Glucose, which is what carbohydrates and protein break down as, burns as sugar and is very inflammatory which adds to an already inflamed condition. Remember, "chronic inflammation is the cause of chronic disease." It makes sense to limit the amount of glucose burning foods you consume.

Now, the problem of burning your stored fat as ketones is that fat cells hold the toxins that we consume over a lifetime and walls them off so they can't harm us. When we burn those stored fats, we risk exposing our bodies to a boatload of these stored toxins. This is why some people get the "keto flu." This is actually your body responding to, and not being able to handle, the toxic load you are releasing while burning your stored fat.

This is a good thing and a bad thing. We do want to get rid of the toxins, but it has to be done correctly

or it can actually make matters worse and make you sick or sicker. In this course, I will walk you through this process.

How to Beat Age-Related Diseases

Age-related disease can be slowed down and even reversed. I mentioned "telomeres" in an earlier chapter, but I didn't go into much detail. Telomeres are little strands or strings attached to the ends of your DNA. Each time a cell divides, as does the DNA, the strand gets a bit shorter. It's kind of like those horsetails that grow by a pond or stream; do you remember breaking them off in sections? Finally, there is nothing left to break off, and so it is with the telomeres. When they reach a certain length, the cells can no longer divide and the cells are supposed to die – I repeat, they are supposed to!

The problem is that, these days, our immune systems are pretty weak, and the other disrupters in our bodies allow these old cells to remain. They become what is called senescent cells, or senile cells; they just take up space and contribute nothing. In fact, they can mutate into cancer cells or just become inflamed and affect the surrounding cells, wreaking havoc in the body. These senescent cells are kind of like bored

teenagers; they are going to cause trouble. As you learn the steps of the Cellular Healing Lifestyle, you will help your body eliminate these unwanted cells.

Heavy Metal Detox

The question isn't, do we have heavy metals? Instead, it is how much do we have, along with a combination of other toxins causing chronic inflammation and turning on bad genes? The best way to know your toxic load is by doing a heavy metal urine challenge test. This is a six-hour collection test. You take a provoking agent just before to help pull the metals out of your tissues and organs, so we get a better reading. Once we know what level of toxicity you have, we can determine what actions to take.

Molds and Hidden Infections

Mold is a tough customer, and it takes hold in and around where heavy metals hide. These molds are alive and have a byproduct called mycotoxins. These can be at the root of many autoimmune conditions. Mold, combined with heavy metals and other opportunistic bugs, like viruses including Lyme and its co-infections, bacteria, etc., like to hole up together in what is often called "hidden infection." These can

be difficult to find but are often at the root of many unresolved health issues.

A comprehensive program with various lab tests can really help nail down why you are not getting well. New information comes out every day and our Health Centers of the Future group is on top of it, sometimes years before the standard medical system embraces it. Even many alternative practitioners are still are slow on the uptake.

At any rate, my goal is to help you understand how to get yourself healthy and keep yourself healthy. Other than the TRT machine and chiropractic adjustments, which have to be done in an office, the rest you can learn and adapt to as your lifestyle changes toward better health!

Fire Your Boss or Other Troublemakers

Don't let others steal your dreams. So many times, clients talk to their would-be friends, and they are talked out of change. Friends claim, "it's for your own good." Even if these people's motives are good, look at their track record. Remember, "If it's to be, it's up to me," and it is!

It has been said that in five years you will be like the people you hang out with and the books you

read. Take a minute and examine this statement regarding your life. Look back and see if it relates to you. It's never too late for a new beginning. There is a whole world out there waiting to meet you.

Feel free to use the two phrases my coach repeated to me time after time, as they helped me tremendously!

1. Nothing's killed you yet.
2. 99.99 percent of the things you worry about never happen.

Additionally, reflect on this phrase: "What you think about, you talk about; what you talk about, you bring about."

I recommend writing these phrases down and sticking them on your bathroom mirror.

I hope you join me and our group of Health Rebels who are taking back our health! Getting healthy should be fun and should not be done alone. There are many sources of great information out there, and new breakthroughs every day. You deserve to be part of the movement!

Thank You!

Welcome to your new life. I encourage you to start again every day. You cannot fail at this process because it is a lifestyle change. Every day, you move a bit closer to a healthier you. There will be setbacks along the way, and you will feel scared that the pain has come back to stay. But don't panic; you know what to do. You've got this!

Your innate power should never be underestimated. Your body has the power to heal, as long as you just get out of its way. Take away any poisons across every side of the health triangle and watch miracles happen.

If you need help, I am a phone call away. Feel free to fill out the neurotoxic questionnaire located at www.mccollumwellness.com. Send it in, and mention

this book so I can offer you a complimentary phone consultation. If I think I can help you, I'll let you know. If I think you would be better served with another practitioner, I will do everything in my power to find the right person to help you!

If you found this information helpful, pass it forward. Let your health legacy begin!

Website: www.mccollumfamilychiropractic.com
Facebook: Dr. Duncan McCollum DC
Private Facebook Group: Health Rebels
Online Classes:

Cellular Healing Lifestyle, 7-Week Intermittent Fasting Keto Lifestyle Class

True Cellular Detox three-month group program

McCollum Family Chiropractic
3555 Clares St. Ste. WW
Capitola, CA, 95010
(831) 459 9990

About the Author

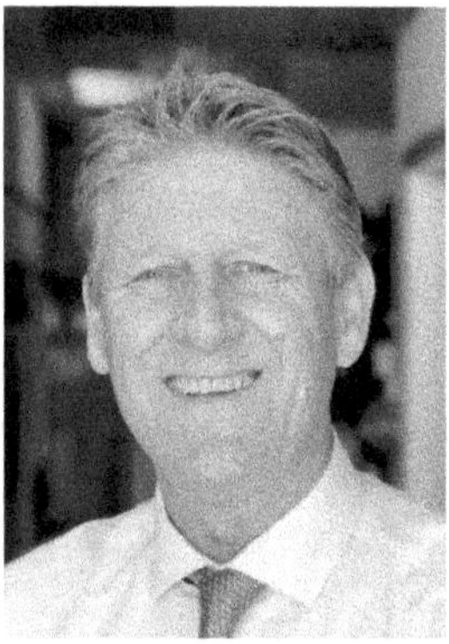

Dr. Duncan McCollum graduated from Palmer College of Chiropractic-West in 1989. He opened his practice that same year and loves serving the Santa Cruz community and now, through the internet, the world. With a strong interest in regenerative health, he continually strives to improve his knowledge on current natural health trends. Dr. McCollum is a sought-after speaker, radio talk show

host, best-selling author, and, for several years, a regenerative and cellular healing teacher.

Three principles in natural healing compel Dr. McCollum to stay on the cutting edge of emerging health science. Those principles are Dr. B.J. Palmer's belief that the body has an innate ability to heal itself from "above, down, inside out;" Dr. Reggie Gold's thought "the body needs no help, it just needs no interference;" and Dr. Dan Pompa's statement of "fix the cell to get well."

As an early adapter of cellular healing. Dr. McCollum finds himself closely aligned with Dr. Dan Pompa, who is considered the world leader in cellular healing. Dr. McCollum teaches the Cellular Healing Lifestyle and has become an expert in the art of cellular detoxification. By combining these principles with his thirty years in the chiropractic field, he has developed remarkable protocols which yield amazing results.

Dr. McCollum understands that the way to a healthy body is through understanding, and he lives by and loves the old adage "Give a man a fish and you feed him for a day. Teach a man to fish and you feed him for a lifetime."

Other Books by Duncan McCollum

The Adventures of Little Big Jim

Coaling Station A

Journey's End

Kaleidoscope

CPSIA information can be obtained
at www.ICGtesting.com
Printed in the USA
JSHW030027180521
14893JS00006B/120

9 781950 367979